ALSO BY EVELINA WEIDMAN STERLING
AND ANGIE BEST-BOSS

Budgeting for Infertility

BEFORE
YOUR TIME

The Early Menopause
Survival Guide

EVELINA WEIDMAN STERLING, Ph.D.
ANGIE BEST-BOSS

A FIRESIDE BOOK
Published by Simon & Schuster

NEW YORK   LONDON   TORONTO   SYDNEY

Fireside
A Division of Simon & Schuster, Inc.
1230 Avenue of the Americas
New York, NY 10020

First Fireside trade paperback edition April 2010

FIRESIDE and colophon are registered trademarks of Simon & Schuster, Inc.

For information about special discounts for bulk purchases, please contact Simon &
Schuster Special Sales at 1-866-506-1949 or business@simonandschuster.com.

The Simon & Schuster Speakers Bureau can bring authors to your live event. For more
information or to book an event contact the Simon & Schuster Speakers Bureau
at 1-866-248-3049 or visit our website at www.simonspeakers.com.

Designed by Ruth Lee-Mui

Manufactured in the United States of America

1 3 5 7 9 10 8 6 4 2

Library of Congress Cataloging-in-Publication Data
Sterling, Evelina Weidman.
Before your time / Evelina Weidman Sterling, Angie Best-Boss.
p. cm.
Includes bibliographical references and index.
1. Menopause—Popular works. I. Best-Boss, Angie. II. Title.
RG186.S746 2010
618.1'75—dc22   2009035800

ISBN 978-1-4391-0845-1
ISBN 978-1-4391-3492-4 (ebook)

Authors' Note

The contents of this work are intended to further understanding and discussion and are not intended to recommend or promote a specific diagnosis or treatment for any person. In light of ongoing research, changes in government regulations, and changes in treatment and diagnostic protocols, the reader is strongly urged to consult with her own health care professionals and to carefully review all medical information.

While publications, Web sites, organizations, and individual practitioners are mentioned in this book, either as citations or as suggested sources of information, the authors do not necessarily endorse all of the information or opinions presented by a provider or organization.

*This book is humbly dedicated to all of the women
who gave deeply of their time and friendship,
sharing their experiences with us
so that others might benefit from their struggles.
We honor you.*

Contents

Part Four: Living Well

Part Five: Looking Ahead

Foreword

Dr. Marcie Richardson

As the baby boomers enter the final third of their lives, menopause has come out of the closet. Bookstores have shelves of books and pharmacies have scores of over-the-counter remedies to help women manage this normal life transition. And that does not even touch upon what is available on the Internet: information, infomercials, propaganda, and products ranging from special sweat-absorbing bedding to vaginal exercisers and hormones of all varieties. Menopause obviously has great meaning for women, but it also generates controversy among scholars, medical experts, and others who write and think about women and their lives. But early menopause is different.

Every year or so, as a generalist in obstetrics and gynecology, I see young women with menstrual irregularities—maybe a few hot flashes, or maybe not. Some might have noticed vaginal dryness. Some will have a mother or sister who went through menopause early. And over the subsequent weeks as testing is completed (it can take some time because some of the testing has to be timed by the menstrual cycle) the diagnosis of premature menopause unfolds. It's not cancer, it isn't really life threatening, but it is devastating to these women.

And then there are the women I see in my Menopause Consultation Clinic, who come in with the diagnosis of premature menopause or premature ovarian failure. Often it has taken months or years to arrive at an explanation for their symptoms. They are often baffled and uninformed—or misinformed. They have low self-esteem, can be depressed, and their relationships are often suffering.

The milestones in a woman's life, of which menopause is one, not only mark the passage of time but also help define her role in society.

Women who don't have normal periods or are infertile or who have premature menopause have a lot to contend with. They have to first understand their condition and get all the medical information available, then they sometimes have to readjust their life expectations and communicate those to the people they know and love. Such women need all the help they can get and are fortunate to have *Before Your Time* as a source of support.

The terms "premature menopause," the bleaker "premature ovarian failure," or the terms that some experts are proposing more recently like "primary ovarian insufficiency" or even "premature ovarian aging" tell a story. Each name tells a different story. It's the story of a natural process happening too soon—sometimes way too soon. Is this condition a "failure" of a woman's ovaries—the organ that makes her female? Does the gentler "insufficiency" help women, or belie the complexity and significance of these conditions? These are the questions that women—and their physicians—are grappling with, and it's among the many that are explored within these pages.

But keep in mind: the medical understanding of early menopause is definitely a work in progress. More is being clarified about the genetic and autoimmune nature of failing ovaries every day, and there is much more to be revealed. The options for fertility treatments or ways to build a family expand all the time. And of course there are the persistent, troubling uncertainties about the harms and benefits of hormone therapy (where most of the data and much of medical and nonmedical opinion derives from studies of women a decade or two older than those with early menopause).

Evelina Weidman Sterling and Angie Best-Boss are accomplished women's health advocates and educators who have both had personal experience with infertility. In this ambitious book they discuss female reproductive physiology and the ways it can go awry and cause early menopause. Then they address the broad implications these conditions have for the health and well-being of the women who find themselves menopausal "before their time." Evelina and Angie have consulted experts and talked with women. And they have brought their own thoughtful perspective to their presentation.

Between 1 and 10 percent of women have ovaries that age early. And then there are women who have their ovaries surgically removed for cancer or other reasons, and the women who have their ovaries damaged by chemotherapy. Early menopause is more common than one might think. If you are one of those women, or know one of those women, you are lucky to have found this book to help you navigate the years ahead. And I am grateful to Evelina and Angie, who have given me something to offer the next patient I see who has had menstrual irregularities, perhaps some hot flashes, elevated FSH, indicating that she is soon to be menopausal.

Readers of this book will gain a framework to understand their medical condition and resources to assist them in getting the care they need going forward. And perhaps most important of all, they will hear the voices of others who share their journey and know they are not alone.

DR. MARCIE RICHARDSON is director of the menopause consultation service and assistant medical director in OB/GYN for clinical quality at Harvard Vanguard Medical Associates, a clinical instructor in obstetrics and gynecology at Harvard Medical School, and practices general OB/GYN at Harvard Vanguard and Beth Israel Deaconess Hospital in Boston. She served on the board of trustees of the North American Menopause Society (NAMS) for nine years, where she sat on the executive committee; and she was past chair of the NAMS Education Committee. For the past fifteen years, she has served on the advisory board of Harvard Women's Health Watch. She was an editorial adviser for the production team of *Our Bodies, Ourselves: Menopause.*

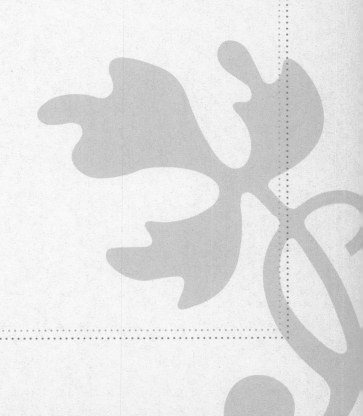

PART ONE

Understanding

What's Going On

1

Not Your Mother's Menopause

*After twenty years of regular monthly reminders that "I am Woman,"
this absence of regularity is somewhat confusing. I am thirty-six,
and part of what makes this tough is that a lot of people outside of
my support network have never heard of this condition [premature
menopause] and don't always realize what I am going through,
emotionally and physically. It feels like getting hit broadside by a
speeding menopause bullet train to Hell, and you're up to your
eyeballs with symptoms that make whacking yourself over the
head with a two-by-four seem like a fun idea. Now what?*

—Leah

MORE THAN SIX THOUSAND women enter menopause each day. For
many, this change of life arrives too suddenly or too soon. Early or
premature menopause results from a wide variety of causes—and is
much more common than you think. Women who suffer from an autoimmune disorder, have survived cancer, undergone a hysterectomy,
been diagnosed with premature ovarian failure, or who just inherited a
bad case of genetics can all experience changes in their ovarian function. More than 5 million women have either experienced early menopause or are at risk for experiencing it.

What's the big deal? There was a musical made about menopause—
how bad can it be? Older women often embrace menopause as an entry
into a new (and sometimes better) phase of life. Think of it: a new sense
of self-assurance, grown kids, no mortgage, increased disposable in-
come, and more free time—who isn't ready for that?

But early menopause doesn't rate the same hoopla. You get lots of the symptoms, none of the perks. And doctors aren't really sure what to do with you. Instead, women are left wondering, "What the hell is going on? This isn't supposed to be happening—not at this age, anyway! What's a girl to do?" This book will help you better understand early menopause (including exactly what it is, why it happens, and what it should be more accurately called) and provide you with the necessary information and skills you need to take control of your life, mind, body, and soul.

Before we embarked on this project, we had many questions ourselves. Searching on the Internet and in bookstores for books on menopause, we were bombarded with images of friendly, older, "grandmotherly" types. You know the pictures—a woman with perfectly coiffed silver hair, usually wearing some pastel shade, either gardening or surrounded by colorful flowers. She is smiling one of those huge smiles that extend ear to ear as if saying "Isn't this grand!" It can be if you're in your fifties and menopause is seen as a badge of honor.

But what about for younger women—what's in it for them? No resources reflected the struggles described by women we knew. We knew there had to be something better. We needed something that would speak to the millions of women who are blindsided by irregular menstrual cycles or early menopause wreaking havoc in their otherwise normal lives. We started asking women's health experts: What are women who go through this supposed to do? Unfortunately, a common response was "menopause is menopause" at any age. But not all women are the same. Most women in their twenties, thirties, or even forties have very little in common with their mother's or grandmother's generations. Why, then, should the experiences be the same?

Our sex lives are different. Changing hormones strain relationships far differently when you are in your thirties than it does for women in their fifties. The treatments aren't the same either. Women have different questions about hormone therapy. What might be safe and appropriate for an older woman to take for a decade or so may not be safe for her daughter to take for forty years or vice versa—what may be recommended for younger women may not be right for older women. Plus, family-building plans are impacted.

Early menopause isn't something we talk about easily with girlfriends. At our age, most women's reproductive cycles run like clockwork. Women may have several friends and colleagues going through the same issues but never know it. More than one woman has kept tampons in her desk drawer so her colleagues won't suspect she isn't "normal." Many women who go through this feel alone.

What Is Normal?

Unlike age-appropriate menopause, which is completely expected and considered a part of the natural aging process, there is nothing normal or natural about early or premature menopause. In fact, using the term "menopause" implies that it's a natural process that is just occurring a little earlier than usual. No big deal, right? Wrong!

The typical age of menopause is around fifty. But for millions of women hormone changes occur before the age of forty. The complete cessation of menstruation that occurs before this age, whether surgically induced (such as after a hysterectomy), medication-induced (after some forms of cancer treatment), or due to plain old luck-of-the-draw genetics, is known as premature menopause. Everything from the environment to premature ovarian failure, cancer, and other illness plays a role, and diminishing ovarian function can actually start at any age.

A few important statistics about premature and early menopause:

- Half a million women go through premature menopause each year because their ovaries stop functioning normally.
- Two million women experience surgical menopause annually.
- More than 60,000 women of childbearing age are diagnosed with some type of cancer annually. Cancer treatments (such as chemotherapy, radiation, and surgery) can all cause early menopause.
- More than 500,000 young women are survivors of childhood cancer or cancer during their early reproductive years; most of them will experience the side effect of early menopause.

When Something Is Wrong

The best decision I have made so far about this condition is this: I made sure I educated myself about my condition. I talked about it with people. When I first found out, I felt very alone; I didn't know that there were other people out there with the same situation. I have also come to some sort of peace with this. It has taken me a long time. I allow myself to cry about it when I feel down about it, but I also reach out when I need help. The good thing is, I know I am not alone.

—Marybeth

We believe you can take charge of both your health and your life. You are unique, and there is no cookie-cutter approach to your health and well-being that will make you instantly happy, perfectly healthy, and rich beyond your wildest dreams. (We wish!) No two women will have exactly the same pattern of symptoms or long-term concerns, so the decisions you make may be different from the decisions someone else with the same diagnosis makes. That doesn't mean you are right and she is wrong or vice versa. It may mean that what you choose to do for treatment is right for *right now.* How you address your health and well-being will likely change over the years, and we hope it does. In this book we give you the tools to take the helm.

A disruption of the menstrual cycle can be a difficult transition for any woman, but when it comes long before you are ready, it can include many additional challenges. However, life can be good while you are living with and adapting to this reproductive system challenge. It is entirely possible for you to maintain your youthfulness and vibrancy and live a very full and satisfying life. It may require counseling, medical treatment, lifestyle changes, and a great support network, but you can be healthy and happy.

But (there's always a "but," isn't there?) it won't happen overnight. Or in two weeks. And it won't happen automatically. Living well even though your ovaries are malfunctioning will take work, effort, and a decision to do so. You aren't alone. Thousands of women have the same struggles, and their voices will join you along the journey.

In this book, we'll explore some of the most common causes of early and premature menopause in more depth, explaining how to get a proper diagnosis. We'll discuss the different treatment options available to alleviate your symptoms and help you live a healthy life. And we'll look forward, at family-planning options and other lifestyle issues that are sure to arise.

> *I have finally discovered there is too little time in life to punish oneself for conditions one cannot control. I have chosen to lead a life in which I am active in the things I can control, as well as accepting the conditions I cannot. I cannot control my primary ovarian insufficiency (POI), but I can control my attitude toward it. I hope to share this attitude with others in the hope that they, too, one day will accept themselves for who they are and not for the disorder they carry. POI is a part of my life, but it is not my life.*
>
> —Carly

2

The Menstrual Cycle
Is a Vital Sign

*Sometimes I wish I could say to all my new dates: "I can't read your
mind, and if you don't envision a future with me, you need to tell me
immediately, no matter how much you're enjoying the sex and/or
companionship. And if we do perchance get married, we're going to
have to work on kids right away. I wish it weren't that way, but
unfortunately it is." Can you imagine his face?*

—Lori

IS IT JUST ME, or is everyone else tired of hearing how famous guys like
David Letterman, Tony Randall, and Larry King can hit one out of the
ballpark despite their advanced paternal age? Larry King was seventy,
for goodness' sake. While contemporary women often have a difficult
enough time getting a grip on the biological clock, ovarian insufficiency
issues bring the biological clock to the foreground.

Back to sex ed for a few minutes. Developing egg cells (oocytes) are
contained in fluid-filled cavities (follicles) in the wall of the ovaries.
Each follicle contains one oocyte. A baby girl is born with egg cells
(oocytes) in her ovaries. Well before we are born (in fact, at about
twenty weeks' gestation), we have about 6 million eggs within our ovaries. Most of them waste away, leaving only 1 to 2 million at birth. By the
time puberty rolls around, we have only about 400,000 eggs left.

Only a small percentage of oocytes mature into eggs. Only a few
hundred (about 500) of these eggs will actually ever be released during

the reproductive years. They are supposed to last us for the rest of our lives; we release only about one every month until they are finally depleted. Until released, an egg remains dormant in its follicle, suspended in the middle of a cell division. Thus, eggs are some of the longest-lived cells in the body. The many thousands of oocytes that do not mature degenerate.

How quickly this depletion occurs is up for debate. Both genetic and environmental factors play an important role, but it is impossible to determine each woman's script. One thing is known: once the eggs are depleted, a woman "officially" enters the time in her life traditionally called menopause. But what exactly does the term "menopause" mean in the context of younger women experiencing this transition?

Literally, menopause is the stopping (or pausing) of your menstrual cycle (or menses). Not all paths to menopause are straightforward and predictable. This process of the ovaries becoming more and more insufficient happens due to a variety of different causes and at various paces. As a result, we like to think of the entire process as more of a continuum rather than a black or white issue, which implies that either you are menopausal or you are not. Obviously, our ovaries are meant to decline naturally from day one and there is nothing anyone can do to stop this process. But once again, we are unclear about what this means and how it affects us as women.

The Biological Clock

We have all heard of the infamous "biological clock." Most often, it goes something like this: you get your first period when you are around twelve to fourteen years old and suddenly become a fertile woman. You then spend the majority of your early couple of decades trying to prevent pregnancy. At some point, you may develop a strong desire to have a baby, so you throw away your birth control, get pregnant, and have a couple of children. You raise these children into adulthood, and if you're lucky, they give you a couple of grandkids. You settle down into retirement, take up mall walking or gardening, and enter menopause. With no children at home, no periods to worry about, and no need for birth control, you enter a new phase of life, feeling freer than you ever have before. After all, isn't this what every happy and healthy woman should aspire to?

Maybe not. It is one version of a life well lived, but not the only one. This type of scenario is not at all accurate or appropriate for all of today's women. Our lives are much too complicated to be tied up into neat little boxes. Some women seek a partner; others don't. Others may not want children or may choose to begin family building after their careers are established.

Our busy lifestyle is erratic at best and does not fit a nice little pre-planned script. Women often struggle to get everything accomplished in a relatively short period of time: finish our education, establish our careers, find the perfect life partner, accumulate some wealth, take care of ourselves, and start our families. Unlike the generations before us, the phases of our lives tend to blur—our twenties, thirties, forties, and fifties meld together without any clear differentiation. Suddenly, thirty is the new twenty, or perhaps fifty is the new thirty? Before we know it, we are left wondering "Where did all the time go?" and, perhaps more important, "How much time do I have left?"

As much as we like to deny it, the biological clock in many ways is still alive and kicking. Biologically speaking, our reproductive organs and abilities are on a deadline and are heavily influenced by the passage of time. We start our periods at a certain time, we can become pregnant at a certain time, and at a certain time we cease being able to reproduce. Unfortunately, we often have little warning about and no control over when these things will happen. Still, every woman is unique. Each of us is influenced by many different factors. In the end, we have no idea about what to expect regarding how our bodies will respond to these many changes.

Despite this uncertainty, we know that our experiences with these transformations are very different from our grandmother's and mother's experiences decades ago. There is no accurate yardstick for women today, nowhere to turn for sage advice from someone wiser. Knowing there is no one else who has walked in our shoes before us, we must find our own way. We are living longer, engaging in a more active lifestyle, enjoying fantastic benefits that only today's society can offer, and confronting new obstacles. We have a lot more knowledge about how our bodies work than ever before. We also have a lot more resources available to address any problems or issues. For the most part, we are no longer viewed as "hysterical" females who have no clue about what is going on with our bodies. We do not have to be passive bystanders anymore. We can be proactive, make decisions for ourselves, and seek out the best treatments that will make us healthier overall.

It's All About the Ovary

The ovary is the linchpin that keeps our menstrual cycle in order. If your menstrual cycle is disrupted, you can assume your ovaries have something to do with it. This seems simple. But unfortunately, many people, including health care professionals, don't seem to get it. When women, no matter what their age, say they have irregular periods, many health care providers offer some simple explanation:

- "Maybe you're just stressed."
- "Try to relax."
- "It's just taking longer for your hormones to even out."
- "All women experience irregular periods, so it's really no big deal."

WHAT IS A "NORMAL" MENSTRUAL CYCLE?

- Girls should start having menstrual periods between the ages of eleven and fourteen. Talk to your doctor if you are over sixteen and haven't had a period yet.
- Cycles should last between twenty-one and thirty-five days.
- Teens may have a little bit more variability, with cycles lasting up to 45 days.
- Bleeding should last between two and seven days from the first day of one period to the first day of the next.
- Normal menstrual flow will require you to use approximately three to six pads or tampons per day.
- While you may experience some pain or cramping, it should not be so severe that it interferes with your everyday activities.

None of these explanations is really on target. The menstrual cycle should be considered a vital sign of good health, the same as your pulse, blood pressure, and temperature. The menstrual cycle is a window into our overall reproductive and general health. In nearly all cases, menstrual cycle disruptions indicate that something else is going on with your body. Exactly what this is varies. It can be a sign of an eating disorder, such as anorexia or bulimia. It can suggest some sort of tumor located somewhere within your endocrine system. It can indicate some type of ovarian disease or be a sign that your ovaries are becoming more and more insufficient.

Whatever the deviation from the "norm," it is essential to get a proper diagnosis as soon as possible so you can treat the root of the problem. The bottom line: irregular periods are not "normal" for any woman. Most women do not experience irregular periods. And for those who do, they are almost always a sign of an underlying medical problem that needs to be addressed.

Too often, health care providers prescribe birth control pills (BCP) for irregular cycles. Oral contraceptives are not a permanent solution for irregular periods. Even worse, BCP will just mask the symptoms so it "appears" everything is working correctly. Whatever was wrong before you started on BCP will remain and sometimes worsen over time. Once you stop the BCP, your symptoms will return, and perhaps much more severely. If this is the case, you will be left with fewer options to deal with your situation most effectively. If you experience irregular cycles or think there is something going on with either your ovulation or your menstrual cycle, it is important to speak up. Don't take "Don't worry about it" or "I see this all the time" as an answer. Do not accept it as "normal."

It is your responsibility to work with your health care provider to figure out what is going on so you can maximize your chances to effectively treat whatever is causing your menstrual cycle changes. Because skipping periods or having delayed periods can be a first indication of other health issues, it's important to be open and honest about your menstruation and note anything abnormal or peculiar.

What Is an Irregular Period?

Most women experience monthly periods anywhere between twenty-eight and thirty-two days apart. However, anything between twenty-one and thirty-five days is considered "regular." Basically, anything outside this range can be considered "irregular." *Oligomenorrhea* refers to infrequent periods with intervals of more than thirty-five days, while *amenorrhea* is the medical term for the absence of a menstrual period among women of reproductive age, usually for at least three months.

So how do you know if something is wrong? First of all, get to know your body and the "normal" rhythm of things. Maybe your periods are becoming increasingly harder and harder to predict. Do you find yourself skipping periods or having longer time intervals between periods? Perhaps you think things have never been "normal" for you when it comes to your period. These could all be signs that something is going on elsewhere in your body that is affecting your menstrual cycle. We have included a monthly menstrual calendar tracker at the end of the book so you can chart your cycle days, as well as any other symptoms you may be experiencing.

Additionally, pay attention to the symptoms of your menstrual cycle. Though all women experience some symptoms as their cycle changes throughout the month, they should not be debilitating or even overly annoying. Look for symptoms such as very heavy blood flow, changes in the overall duration of your periods, breakthrough bleeding between periods, severe pain or cramps at any time during your cycle, excess bloating, emotional symptoms, or difficulty concentrating. Any of these symptoms could be a sign of other health issues.

Uncovering the Cause

When you go to see your health care provider because you're not having periods, she will want to learn where the problem lies. For example, is it in your hypothalamus, the pituitary, the ovary, or in the uterus? To begin to sort out the problem that's keeping you from having a menstrual cycle, your health care provider will probably give you a series of tests to measure your hormones, especially FSH, or follicle-stimulating hormone (we'll learn more about this hormone and these tests in Chapter 3).

Dr. Lawrence Nelson, an expert on the menstrual cycle at the National Institutes of Health, compares the hypothalamus to a thermostat. It measures the temperature, and the ovaries are kind of like a furnace. The furnace and the thermostat together form a "feedback system," as do the hypothalamus, pituitary, and ovaries. If your thermostat senses that the temperature in the room is too low, it sends a signal to the furnace to turn on and make heat to raise the temperature.

What happens when the temperature in the room gets too high? It sends a signal to the furnace to turn off and stop making heat; then the temperature falls a little bit and the furnace comes on and makes heat to get it up again. This is called a feedback control system. To keep the temperature in a narrow range, the thermostat and the furnace regulate the room temperature by turning the furnace on and off.

"A similar feedback system works with the hypothalamus and the ovary, with regard to estrogen. If the estrogen level is low, the hypothalamus sends a signal; these follicles grow and make estrogen," Nelson explains. "That raises the level of estrogen in the blood, and then the hypothalamus senses that this level of estrogen in the blood is enough, so it sends the signal to the pituitary for FSH, so if the ovary can't respond, the FSH level is going to be high, because it's going to keep sending the signal harder and harder to try to get the ovary to work."

A doctor can thus tell if the problem is in the hypothalamus, pituitary, or ovary by measuring hormone levels. For example, if the FSH level is high, that means things are working okay in the brain, and it's trying to send a signal to the ovary to get it to make estrogen; thus the problem is in the ovary and the ovary's not responding. Once your health care provider understands why your periods are irregular, you will have a better understanding of what is happening with your body.

Ovarian Insufficiency or Menopause?

Unless you experience surgically or medically induced menopause (which we will discuss later), the steps toward ovarian insufficiency (sometimes called early menopause, though, as you'll see below, this term isn't quite accurate) occur much more gradually. In fact, the symptoms can be so subtle that at first you may not even notice that you are starting to go through changes. For most women, this transition occurs over the span of several years. But depending on your circumstances, it can be anywhere between zero to ten years in duration. Overall, the experience is not a linear progression but rather a continuum most women cycle into and out of before ovulation ceases.

Since your hormones fluctuate gradually, it is possible that you will move back and forth between some of these steps before settling down into one specific phase. Also, it is difficult to know how long you will be at any one step before you move to the next. Therefore, it is important for you to understand your hormones and know how they are affecting you. If you remain aware of your hormones and related symptoms throughout your life, you will be able to notice any changes or trends that may be occurring.

STEP ON THE GAS

Dr. Richard Sherbahn of the Advanced Fertility Center of Chicago describes FSH this way:

> Think of it like stepping on the gas pedal in the car to get going. The FSH is the gas, and the pituitary gland releases FSH to get a follicle "going" at the beginning of every menstrual cycle. If there are less follicles left, and perhaps lower-quality follicles, the amount of "gas" has to be increased to get a follicle developing. In a menopausal woman, the gas pedal is on the floor for the rest of her life, even though there are no follicles or eggs left. The woman's body never gives up trying; FSH levels are permanently elevated.

HIGH FOLLICLE-STIMULATING HORMONE LEVELS

Usually women don't have a clue about ovulation until they try to become pregnant. Most often, FSH levels are tested when a woman is trying to become pregnant and having no success. High FSH levels can indicate that your eggs are too few and of too low a quality to become pregnant. "You have a high FSH level" is usually the first indication a woman hears when experiencing some aspect of ovarian insufficiency.

FSH levels vary widely, so don't make any assumptions (good or bad) based on only one test. Have the test repeated over the course of several months (or several cycles) to get a more accurate picture. Also, FSH readings can vary among labs. FSH is complex, and it is often difficult to get an accurate reading. Keep this in mind when you are looking at several readings or are considering seeing a new doctor. You shouldn't "officially" consider yourself as having high FSH unless you have had several FSH tests across several cycles that all indicate elevated FSH levels.

Still, it is difficult to know how quickly your FSH levels will continue to increase. While not 100 percent accurate, age is probably the strongest predictor. If you are older (in your midthirties or forties), the likelihood of your FSH increasing faster is greater than if you are younger (in your twenties). Although it is more common in your midthirties to forties, high FSH levels can start occurring at any age. Regardless, time is a critical factor in addressing high FSH levels. The sooner you know and understand your FSH levels, the better off you will be. And the earlier you are diagnosed with high FSH levels, the more options you will have if you want to become pregnant.

GRADE-A EGGS

It's not enough to have eggs; you need good ones. Poor egg quality can mean that:

- Eggs do not implant into the uterine wall after fertilization.
- Eggs implant but cannot grow due to insufficient energy.
- There is a greater likelihood of abnormal chromosomes; any children born may have genetic abnormalities, such as Down syndrome.

"In general, your ovarian reserve is as bad as your worst FSH. If you have an FSH of fifteen in one cycle and then a seven in another cycle, the situation is not improving. Some women 'bounce around' with FSH levels in the normal to abnormal range. However, they tend to respond and have chances for pregnancy as predicted by their highest FSH level. Waiting for a menstrual cycle with a lower FSH level and then stimulating right away for in vitro fertilization (IVF) is not of any proven benefit," Dr. Sherbahn explains.

All women, even young ones, experience changes in FSH levels, and this continues throughout life. There is still a lot we don't know about these fluctuations because most women do not have this hormone checked regularly. Not surprisingly, our data on this topic are therefore severely skewed. With such a limited population from which to draw, the assumption is made that if you have high FSH levels you will automatically have difficulty becoming pregnant and experience related symptoms as your ovaries begin to fail.

In actuality, this may not always be the case. Given the lack of scientific evidence, we don't fully understand FSH fluctuations and how these changes really affect women. The truth of the matter is that there are probably millions of women with higher-than-normal FSH levels who experience no symptoms at all, have fairly regular periods, and are able to become pregnant without any assistance. Even a small percentage (usually between 5 and 10 percent) of women with documented high FSH levels conceive spontaneously. But these are not the women who seek care and have their hormone levels checked. Therefore, little research has been done on this topic, which leaves many critical questions unanswered, including:

- What exactly is a normal FSH level?
- How many women are affected by high FSH levels?
- Why does FSH affect women differently?
- At what point does FSH start contributing to problems?

PRIMARY OVARIAN INSUFFICIENCY (POI) AND PREMATURE OVARIAN FAILURE (POF)

For many women who have higher-than-normal FSH levels, their ovaries eventually begin to be affected, causing a number of menopause-like symptoms. Both primary ovarian insufficiency (POI) and premature ovarian failure (POF) are terms used rather interchangeably to describe when the ovaries begin to stop functioning normally in women younger than age forty.

Because this can be a long process, POI is the preferred term; it more accurately portrays the gradual loss of ovarian functioning over the course of years. On the other hand, POF implies a complete or nearly complete ovarian "failure" in women younger than age forty. Since actual ovarian "failure" is rare among women with these symptoms, we prefer the more accurate description POI.

Because POI is so difficult to diagnosis and is severely underdiagnosed, it is not clear how many women are affected. Estimates suggest somewhere between 1 and 4 percent of women have POI. More specifically:

- 1 in 100 women will have POI by age forty.
- 1 in 250 women will have POI by age thirty-five.
- 1 in 1,000 women will have POI by age thirty.
- 1 in 10,000 women will have POI by age twenty.

Adding to the confusion is the fact that although POI is considered a disease related to the menstrual cycle, its diagnosis is often not definitive. Insufficient ovarian function can alternate with normal ovarian function and menstrual cycles returning intermittently, allowing natural pregnancies to occur occasionally even after a POI diagnosis. Not all women experience the same symptoms, which makes it nearly impossible to know exactly how many women are affected.

It is important to note that POI is *not* menopause. Menopause is a naturally occurring event that happens to women at age fifty-one on average. POI is not a natural life event and strikes women at age twenty-seven on average. POI can occur in adolescents as young as fourteen years old and in women as old as thirty-nine. Menopause is the permanent cessation of menstruation; with POI, women can sometimes still experience spontaneous ovarian activity and periods. In fact, up to 25 percent of women diagnosed with POI still have viable follicles and ovulate periodically. Moreover, about 5 to 10 percent of these women do become pregnant on their own without any assisted reproductive technologies.

POI should be considered as a continuum of disorders, as follows:

- "Occult POI" is a condition in which a woman still has regular menstrual cycles and a normal blood level of FSH but POI is diagnosed on the basis of otherwise unexplained infertility (which can be associated with poor egg quality) or a low ovarian response to fertility medications.
- "Biochemical POI," which is diagnosed on the basis of an elevated blood level of FSH, may also be accompanied by infertility.
- "Overt POI" is a condition in which women have an elevated blood level of FSH in association with irregular menstrual cycles, sometimes accompanied by other typical symptoms such as hot flashes. This is the most advanced clinical problem and is characterized by a complete absence of eggs, although it is not actually possible to prove that there are no eggs in the ovaries.

Women do not necessarily progress through these different conditions in a linear fashion. In other words, women may have biochemical POI (elevated blood FSH), then develop overt POI (irregular cycles), then experience a return to regular cycles for some time.

Diminished Ovarian Reserve (DOR)

As a woman ages, her fertility decreases, especially the number of good-quality eggs she has left. This decrease occurs slowly up until about age thirty-five, when it falls even faster—a major reason women have more difficulty becoming pregnant as they get older. This drop in fertility is seen even among women who have perfectly normal and regular menstrual cycles. Diminished ovarian reserve is a natural part of the aging process and is not considered primary ovarian insufficiency. Unlike POI, women with DOR do not experience the other symptoms associated with changing hormone levels. Infertility is the primary concern.

Early or Premature Menopause

While most women who have POI/POF will continue to menstruate sporadically, the term "menopause" means the total cessation of your period. Most women go through menopause sometime between forty-five and fifty-five. In general, early or premature menopause refers to the timing of ovarian insufficiency. In *early menopause,* periods completely cease earlier than usual, typically before age forty-five. However, even women well into their forties consider it too early to experience menopause. Women are living longer and many are waiting longer to build their families, so they do not consider that they are entering the menopausal age even when they reach the so-called normally accepted age range.

Premature menopause usually refers to women under age forty who stop menstruating completely. In this case, it is often not premature menopause but rather POI, since most women will still have an occasional and unpredictable cycle. Both POI and premature menopause are extremely difficult to diagnose because most health care providers do not consider irregular menstrual cycles as a serious concern, particularly outside fertility concerns. Regardless, an unexpected disruption of one's reproductive cycle can be devastating for women at any age.

Ovarian insufficiency can occur suddenly as the result of surgery or medical treatments. For other women, it occurs more gradually and might be attributed to family history. To determine if you are at higher risk for early menopause, look at when your own mother or other close female relatives started to go through menopause. Even though there are no guarantees, it is likely that you will follow a similar schedule. Similarly, some research suggests that smoking leads to menopause two years earlier than average. If you have never had children, you are more likely to experience menopause at an earlier age.

WHAT'S THE DIFFERENCE?
A woman in menopause has virtually no chance of getting pregnant on her own because her periods have completely stopped. A woman with ovarian insufficiency has a greatly reduced chance of getting pregnant, but pregnancy is still possible because she does get her period occasionally.

Perimenopause

Even this early transition to menopause is not clear-cut. Perimenopause marks the time period in which your body is beginning its transition into menopause. Perimenopause encompasses the years leading up to menopause, when you completely stop getting your period. It can last anywhere from two to eight years, including the first year after your final period. If "normal" menopause falls anywhere between forty-five and fifty-five, it is quite possible that you might begin to experience some of the effects of perimenopause in your midthirties.

Perimenopause involves hormone levels rising and falling unevenly. As a result, you will experience many of the same symptoms of menopause. Women wonder whether they are actually experiencing menopause and how long perimenopause will last before their reproductive capacity is gone.

RACIAL AND ETHNIC DIFFERENCES

Women across all races and ethnicities experience variations with regard to ovarian insufficiency and premature menopause. However, some research has suggested that these types of disruptions in ovarian function may be more prevalent among Caucasian, African-American, and Latina women, especially compared to women of Asian origin, such as Chinese and Japanese. Because how women respond to certain menopause-related symptoms also varies by culture, women may report different symptoms associated with ovarian insufficiency and early menopause.

Not all women are the same, nor are their experiences with ovarian insufficiency. This is an important area to explore further so we can obtain more answers and figure out this complicated puzzle, such as which factors have the most influence in decreasing ovarian function.

Secondary Ovarian Insufficiency

While primary ovarian insufficiency is the result of ovaries that are not working properly, secondary ovarian insufficiency is the result of a temporarily inadequate or inappropriate function of ovaries. This is often referred to as amenorrhea, which is the absence of a period for several months. Unlike POI, in which women must struggle with insufficient ovarian function and cessation of periods throughout their lives, women who experience secondary ovarian insufficiency will have their ovarian function and cycles restored once the cause of the problem is identified and treated. As we have discussed before, once you start experiencing irregular periods, it is important to have it checked out. It can be the result of a number of causes, which need to be ruled out before a diagnosis of primary ovarian insufficiency or early menopause is given. Some of these other causes include the following.

POLYCYSTIC OVARY SYNDROME (PCOS)

PCOS is one of the most common causes of irregular periods, affecting as many as 10 percent of women worldwide. PCOS is caused by an imbalance in the hormones that communicate between the pituitary gland, located at the base of the brain, and the ovaries. In general, PCOS happens when luteinizing hormone (LH) and/or insulin levels are too high, combined with extra testosterone being produced by the ovary. It usually starts at puberty; other common symptoms include unwanted hair on the face or other parts of the body, acne, weight gain and/or trouble losing weight, patches of dark skin on the back of the neck or other areas (called acanthosis nigricans), sleep apnea, and ovarian cysts.

PCOS is diagnosed through blood tests and an ultrasound of the uterus and ovaries. While there is no cure for PCOS, it can be effectively managed. Many women have success though maintaining a healthy lifestyle including good nutrition and daily exercise. There are also excellent long-term medications to help manage the symptoms, including hormone treatment and insulin-sensitizing medications. It is critical to diagnose and treat PCOS properly because like ovarian insufficiency, it can affect fertility as well as put a woman at higher risk for developing depression, diabetes, cardiovascular disease, and other long-term health problems.

CONGENITAL ADRENAL HYPERPLASIA (CAH)

Congenital adrenal hyperplasia refers to a group of inherited disorders of the adrenal gland. Usually diagnosed at birth, girls with CAH fail to menstruate or experience abnormal menstrual periods. Other symptoms may include a deep voice, early appearance of pubic and armpit hair, and excessive hair growth and facial hair. Also, these girls tend to be tall as children and shorter than normal as adults. Treatment with cortisol helps return hormone levels to normal.

Occasionally, the symptoms of CAH occur much later in life. This is known as nonclassical or late-onset CAH. The most common symptoms of late-onset CAH include early age of first menstrual period, menstrual irregularities, thinning hair, and excessive facial hair growth. Because the symptoms are so similar, sometimes women with late-onset CAH are mistakenly diagnosed with PCOS. However, a single blood test assessing adrenal steroid levels, such as 17-hydroxyprogesterone, can provide an accurate diagnosis for late-onset CAH. Overall, Ashkenazi Jews, Italians, and Hispanics have higher rates of late-onset CAH than the general population.

HYPERPROLACTINEMIA

Hyperprolactinemia is the presence of abnormally high levels of prolactin in the blood. Prolactin is a hormone produced by the pituitary gland that is associated primarily with lactation. Too much prolactin can disrupt the menstrual cycle. Hyperprolactinemia is most often caused by diseases affecting the pituitary gland (usually a benign tumor). Prolactin levels can also be influenced by prescription drugs, medicinal herbs, or heavy metals. Hyperprolactinemia is diagnosed through blood tests and an MRI to provide images of the pituitary gland. If a tumor is found, it can often be treated effectively with medications such as bromocriptine. Once controlled, prolactin levels return to normal and ovulation and menstruation resume.

Uterine Abnormalities

Uterine abnormalities such as fibroids, cysts, polyps, or endometriosis can cause problems with periods and ovulation. Sometimes these problems might take the form of very frequent, painful, and heavy bleeding. At other times, periods come with no predictable pattern. In either case, it is important to be checked whenever you experience these symptoms or your periods become irregular.

Other Factors

NUTRITION, EXERCISE, AND WEIGHT

Some women's bodies are very sensitive to lifestyle issues such as nutrition and exercise. Poor nutrition, especially a diet too high in carbohydrates, can affect hormone levels. Excessive weight gain or obesity can disrupt hormones and ovulation. Likewise, extreme dieting or low body weight will interrupt many hormonal functions, temporarily halting ovulation. Too much exercise can contribute to irregular periods (missed periods are common among endurance athletes). If you think your lifestyle may be contributing to irregular cycles, talk to your doctor about making appropriate changes. Usually, once the issues related to physical stress, body fat, and high energy expenditure are resolved, menstruation and ovulation return to normal.

MEDICATIONS

Practically anything you put into your body has the potential to affect your hormones. Prescription medications such as antidepressants, blood pressure pills, steroids, antibiotics, and of course birth control pills (along with any other medication that contains hormones) can affect your periods. Some types of oral contraceptives limit the number of times per year that you have a menstrual cycle. Even once you stop taking birth control pills, it may take a couple of months to resume regular ovulation and menstruation. Contraceptives that are injected or implanted such as Depo-Provera or Mirena can stop periods altogether and cause them to become irregular even after the medication is stopped. If you are taking any type of medication (prescription or over the counter), you should have the medication-menstruation connection looked into by your health care provider.

SMOKING AND OTHER DRUG USE

Smoking and many other types of drug use can also contribute to menstrual irregularities. Monthly periods may stop or become irregular, and there is some evidence that tobacco and other drugs may destroy eggs in the ovaries, even among young women. Therefore, the ability to become pregnant may end at an earlier age.

PREGNANCY AND BREAST FEEDING

Because pregnancy and breast feeding cause drastic changes in hormone levels, ovulation and menstruation may be disrupted for up to several months. If you have not exclusively breast-fed in several months and your regular periods have not yet returned, it is important to discuss it with your health care provider and look into other causes.

ILLNESSES AND STRESS

Whenever your body is taxed by physical or emotional stress, it can impact your hormones. Too much stress can result in huge hormone fluctuations, leading to disrupted ovulation and menstruation. However, this is often used as a catch-all explanation for women's menstrual irregularities. It is important to know that while the stress–hormone relationship may seem logical, there have been no conclusive studies looking at the impact of stress on a woman's cycles. Many women who experience tremendous amounts of stress still have fairly normal periods. If you feel you are under stress, try to deal with it effectively. Though some illnesses, especially chronic or long-term ones, can interfere with regular menstruation, menstruation typically resumes as you recover. But if your periods don't return to a normal rhythm within a reasonable time frame, don't continue using it as an excuse or allow a medical professional to do so. It is crucial to consider other possible causes sooner rather than later.

ENVIRONMENTAL TOXINS

Given our society's current interest in the environment, many researchers have suggested a link between environmental toxins and the disruption of menstrual cycles. This makes sense, but unfortunately there is still a lot we don't know. Hopefully more information will become available as more research is conducted. If you have a known history of exposure to environmental toxins, such as in your place of employment, it is probably a good idea to mention it to your doctor as you try to figure out the cause of your menstrual irregularities.

What's at Stake

All in all, a thorough exam needs to be conducted whenever menstrual irregularities are experienced. You and your health care provider should never jump to conclusions based on a single symptom or lab test. Any irregularities in menstruation should be looked at in terms of your overall health and well-being. Ignoring seemingly minor health problems can lead to significantly greater ones later on.

3

Know Your Hormones

For those of you who have gone from doctor to doctor and taken one ineffective medication after another, I think the answer may be to learn as much as possible about your own body and how it works. I wasted so much time believing that the next doctor or naturopath was going to have the perfect answer. They all had a part of the truth, but I had to separate the wheat from the chaff. It's really too bad we don't get an owners' manual to tell us more, but we can learn by reading and discussing and sharing our success stories.

—Jill

WE NEED HORMONES TO LIVE. Hormones are what make women, well, women. We have all felt the effects of hormones and probably have even blamed our hormones once or twice when we were feeling a little off. Society has even played into the power of hormones by telling us we are often at their mercy. In fact, we've all heard people say, "Don't listen to her—it's just her hormones talking!"

Jokes about hormones, especially surrounding PMS and menopause, are, unsurprisingly, generally written by men from the "victim's" point of view, and we've all heard them. What does PMS really stand for? Pass My Shotgun, Psychotic Mood Shift, Pack My Stuff, Provide Me with Sweets, Pardon My Sobbing, and Pass My Sweatpants.

Then there's the old favorite, "How many women with PMS [or menopause] does it take to screw in a lightbulb?"

ONE! And do you know WHY it takes only ONE? Because no one

else in this house knows HOW to change a lightbulb. They don't even know the bulb is BURNED OUT. They would sit in this house in the dark for THREE DAYS before they figured it OUT!

Even if you haven't been plagued by hormone problems, you probably know what it's like to feel as though you're being held hostage by your hormones. They are a powerful force in our bodies and affect us physically, emotionally, and mentally. Still, hormones remain shrouded in mystery. Exactly what are they? And how do they affect us, especially at this point in our lives? The more we understand about our hormones and how they affect our body, mind, and emotions, the better we can minimize their negative effects and enhance their positive ones.

What Are Hormones?

Hormones make up one of the body's great communication networks. A hormone is a microscopic molecule released by a gland that travels though the blood until it reaches a cell with a receptor that fits. Similar to a key in a lock, this molecule attaches to the receptor and sends a signal inside the cell. This signal gives certain instructions to the cell, such as to produce a certain protein or start multiplying. Hormones are involved with just about every biological process, including immune function, reproduction, and growth, as well as control of other hormones. Hormones are extremely potent; it doesn't take much to have an impact. Very small amounts of hormones can wreak havoc on your body. Whenever hormones are askew, our body faces consequences.

If a hormone is not working right, or if you have too much or too little of a hormone, it can confuse your body's signaling system. Instead of doing its job, the signal from your body's hormones to the cell is disrupted, and your body is unable to function properly.

While hormones contribute to many biological processes, such as growth, heart rate, and hunger, it is the "sex" hormones that we hear most about. Men and women have all the same sex hormones but in varying amounts. These hormones control and maintain our reproductive systems. They also influence the muscle mass, strength, and behavior of men and women, making us look or act "male" or "female."

Female Sex Hormones

As women age, it is the female reproductive hormones that are affected the most. When a woman's body and reproductive cycle begin to change, her ovaries become less functional. This results in the production of lower levels of hormones; thus the natural rhythm of her reproductive cycle is disrupted. This changes the way a woman's body acts in a number of ways, from mood swings to libido to dry skin and gum disease.

ALL ABOUT ESTROGEN

Though both men and women have estrogen flowing throughout their bodies, estrogens are usually present at significantly higher levels in women, especially during their reproductive years. The term "estrogen" refers to a group of chemically similar hormones found in women, including estradiol (the most abundant), estrone, and estriol. Overall, estrogen is produced primarily in the ovaries, adrenal glands, and fat tissues.

Estrogen has a lot of important functions. First of all, it promotes the development of female secondary sex characteristics, such as breasts, the thickening of the uterine lining, and other aspects of regulating the menstrual cycle. Estrogen is what makes us women. Additionally, it plays a part in growth, metabolism, muscle mass, vaginal lubrication, sex drive, and bone formation. It also contributes to a woman's mental health. Sudden changes in estrogen levels can result in significant mood lowering, leading to feelings of depression.

Because the onset of diminishing ovarian function hits the ovaries hard and the ovaries alone are responsible for about 90 percent of estrogen production, estrogen levels begin to fluctuate a lot more at this time. In most cases (except when they are surgically removed), the ovaries do not turn off smoothly—they sputter. This phase of up-and-down estrogen levels can last for five years or more. Symptoms include hot flashes, irregular menstrual cycles, breast tenderness, exacerbation of migraines, urinary stress incontinence, and mood swings. By the time a woman stops having periods, she is producing only about 40 to 60 percent of the estrogen she produced before her ovarian function began to diminish.

LH AND FSH

Luteinizing hormone (LH) and follicle-stimulating hormone (FSH) are called gonadotropins because they stimulate the gonads—the testes in males and the ovaries in females. While LH and FSH are not necessary to live, they are needed for reproduction. For women, LH induces the ovaries to produce mature follicles, which contain eggs. FSH stimulates the maturation of these follicles (tiny cysts on the ovary). Too much FSH results in "superovulation," or the development of more than the usual number of mature follicles and hence an increased number of eggs. The phenomenon is responsible for becoming pregnant with multiples.

As women age or ovarian function is diminished, FSH levels begin to rise, causing changes in menstrual cycle, irregular cycles, and other menopause-type symptoms. Eventually, this diminishes the ability of the ovaries to produce enough eggs. This rise in FSH continues until well after periods have completely stopped. LH levels also rise during this period, but to a much lesser extent than FSH levels. Unfortunately, it is difficult to measure these hormone changes, since their levels vary considerably in the same individual.

THE PROGESTERONE FACTOR

A great amount of the attention paid to hormones and ovarian insufficiency centers on estrogen. However, progesterone also has important functions that should not be neglected. Progesterone is considered to be the pregnancy (get it? *pro-gestation*) hormone and is responsible for the maturation of the uterine lining needed to receive and sustain a pregnancy. Miscarriages can result if progesterone levels are insufficient. Still, the importance of progesterone does not stop here. Some research has suggested that it plays a role in other body systems, including the urinary tract, heart, blood vessels, bones, skin, hair, mucous membranes, and brain.

WHAT ABOUT TESTOSTERONE?

When we think of testosterone, we usually envision men and their male hormones. But women need testosterone too (much lower levels, of course). Testosterone is naturally produced by the ovaries and the adrenal glands. As ovarian function begins to diminish, many women start to produce less testosterone. In fact, even in "normal" circumstances, by age forty most women produce about half the amount of testosterone they did in their twenties. When menopause-type symptoms happen earlier in life, these levels can drop off sooner and more quickly. Many researchers believe that the diminished energy, decreased sexual desire, and overall "flatness" of mood that some women experience around the time that ovarian function begins to diminish are directly related to declining levels of testosterone. Some researchers even suggest that inappropriate levels of testosterone can contribute to insulin resistance, a precursor to diabetes and cardiovascular disease.

OTHER IMPORTANT HORMONES

Though they aren't officially considered "sex" hormones, there are a couple of others that can affect your overall hormonal balance if left unchecked. Both thyroid-stimulating hormone (TSH) and cortisol are somewhat related to diminished ovarian function. Thyroid hormones are needed to keep everything in order, connected, and communicating in virtually all areas of your body. The thyroid also manages all metabolic functions from appetite to how your food is digested to weight gain. When your thyroid function is out of whack, this severely affects how the rest of your body functions as well.

Cortisol, produced in the adrenal glands, is another vital hormone that helps you handle stress. The adrenal glands are important because they serve as a backup for producing estrogen and progesterone as you get older or your ovarian function begins to wane. Problems with cortisol production can cause depression, memory loss, lack of energy, weight gain, overall aches and pains, and a plethora of other negative effects.

Hormones and Your Menstrual Cycle

Hormones control the menstrual cycle, which is a complicated and perfectly timed series of events. As mentioned before, though most women menstruate every 28 to 32 days, a "normal" menstrual cycle is anywhere between twenty-one and thirty-five days. Anything outside this range is considered abnormal. Unfortunately, the menstrual cycle is one of the most underappreciated and misunderstood biological processes in the human body. Most women are not taught to track their menstrual cycles, so it is often difficult for them to notice changes and know when to discuss them with their health care providers. If you haven't already done so, get to know your menstrual cycle. Understand how your body works. Take any changes seriously, and talk to your health care providers about any changes you notice.

The simplest method to chart your cycle (if you have one) is to count the days and record them on a calendar or chart of some sort. On the day your period starts, you write down on your chart "Day 1: Bleeding." At the next period you do the same thing. This is the most basic form of charting. Day 1 of a woman's cycle is the first full day of menstrual bleeding. Once the uterine lining has built up, it must be shed in order to prepare for the next cycle. Hormone levels drop drastically, causing menstruation to occur.

During the next fourteen days or so, called the follicular phase, the body prepares for ovulation. The pituitary gland releases FSH, which stimulates the follicles within the ovaries to grow and produce an egg. At the same time, the pituitary gland releases LH, which stimulates the follicles to manufacture and secrete estrogen. This estrogen makes the uterine lining build up in order to receive an embryo if the egg is fertilized.

As ovulation is about to occur, LH levels increase even more to stimulate the release of the egg. About twenty-four to thirty-six-hours after this increased LH production, the follicle ruptures and the egg is released into the fallopian tubes, where it can be fertilized. The rest of the ruptured follicle, called the corpus luteum, starts to shrivel up and begins to produce progesterone, a hormone necessary to sustain a pregnancy. Progesterone also helps the endometrium thicken and become more vascular, and in this way the endometrial lining becomes like a "soft pillow" to catch a descending blastocyst (fertilized egg). Then progesterone sends a signal to your brain *not* to commence with menstruation, the shedding of the uterine lining.

The next phase of the menstrual cycle is called the luteal phase and lasts, on average, fourteen days, before your period begins. A short luteal phase is associated with fertility problems. If the egg is fertilized within twenty-four hours of being released, an embryo begins to develop and travel toward the uterus for implantation. If this is the case, progesterone production is increased. If fertilization does not occur, the production of progesterone is slowed. The insufficient supply of progesterone causes the uterine lining to slough off, and another menstrual cycle begins.

Hormones and Diminishing Ovarian Function

Most of us spend our lives thinking that menopause will begin sometime in our fifties, give or take a few years. We also anticipate that this decline in hormone levels will occur gradually, over a period of several years, which should give us time to prepare and ask questions about how this change will affect us. Each year, however, tens of thousands of women between the ages of fifteen and forty-four experience a sudden change in hormone levels, which leaves them floundering in the face of diminishing ovarian function. In this case, changes can occur in a matter of months or even weeks, and they are left wondering "What is happening to me?"

During this time, your hormones are participating in a vicious cycle: A lack of estrogen means the production of LH does not get stimulated. The malfunction in LH stimulation means an egg is not released, which prevents the corpus luteum from releasing the progesterone that would increase the amount of LH and FSH. Of course, this further inhibits the manufacturing of estrogen. And in the end, estrogen can seem to be as important as oxygen, as low levels of it are the root cause of a number of physical and emotional changes.

Hormone Testing

Many young women never think to get their hormones checked. Unless we're trying to get pregnant, we don't think about them much. And frankly, a missed period here and there can seem like a good thing. Granted, the occasional surprise period makes for no fun, but it's not a big deal, either.

Hormone levels are constantly changing throughout our lives. In order to establish a baseline and understand your personal hormone fluctuations, it is important to get your hormone levels checked periodically, starting as soon as you start to notice any problems. Many health care professionals and researchers are encouraging women to get their hormone levels checked if they start to experience menstrual irregularities or have difficulty getting pregnant. If you are still getting your period, it is best to have your hormone levels checked on day three of your menstrual cycle. If you are no longer having periods, you can have them checked at any time.

Types of Hormone Tests

Getting a hormone level screen is essential to get the full picture of what's happening with your body.

BLOOD HORMONE TESTS

Assessing hormones through a blood test is considered the gold standard. A blood hormone test is pretty simple. A single blood sample is taken and sent to a lab for analysis. The blood test needs to be ordered by a licensed medical professional, and several hormones can be tested with just one sample. Blood tests are also usually covered by insurance, and are the most reliable method by far. Ideally, a number of hormone level tests can be performed over a period of time, so comparisons can be made.

SALIVA HORMONE TESTS

Most insurance companies consider salivary tests of estrogen, progesterone, testosterone, melatonin, or dehydroepiandrosterone (DHEA) experimental and investigational for the screening, diagnosis, or monitoring of menopause or diseases related to aging or any other indications, because they have not been proven to be valid alternatives to blood tests. What this means is that they won't pay for them. The North American Menopause Society has concluded, "Salivary testing is not considered to be a reliable measure of hormone levels." And at $300 to $400 each, paying out of pocket for less reliable results isn't a bargain.

Hormone Results

Getting your hormones checked can contribute to an early diagnosis. Knowing about problems early on can sometimes help you control, slow, or even reverse your hormone changes before additional complications occur. Still, it is important to remember that different labs use different values for "normal." As a result, it is sometimes difficult for health care providers to determine exactly where you fall on the hormone range. What might be considered "normal" by one lab might be "abnormal" for another. As a woman, it is essential for you to become an active participant in your own health care and understand your hormones. You know your body best. You need to keep track of any changes that occur and talk with your clinician about these issues.

Any variation with ovarian function is complex. Don't let anyone tell you that you are in menopause or even heading toward menopause based on a single test result. It is more complicated than that, and more attention should be paid to a variety of factors, including test results, your family history, and a description of your symptoms. In terms of diminishing ovarian function or early menopause, the two most important hormones to start with are FSH and estrogen.

AT-HOME HORMONE TESTING

There are also several "at-home" FSH tests. These tests basically involve peeing on a stick. Much like ovulation predictor tests, they involve a stick with two lines; one is the control line, and one is the test line. If the test line is as dark as or darker than the control line, your FSH may be elevated. Even if you are tempted, don't rely on these tests completely. There is too much variability to trust them (not to mention that they are incredibly difficult to read and interpret). If you have any concerns about your menstrual cycle, you are much better off going to a lab and having your blood drawn.

FSH

FSH is probably considered the most important hormone indicating whether your ovarian function is becoming insufficient. It is also used as a rough gauge of ovarian reserve, or how many good-quality eggs you have left. Basically, the closer you are to menopause (or the complete cessation of your menstrual cycle), the fewer good-quality eggs you have left. FSH levels change throughout the menstrual cycle, so it is important to pay attention to what day in your menstrual cycle your FSH level was checked.

Typical normal values of FSH are usually somewhere between 3 and 20 mIU/ml. From a fertility perspective, anything under 6 indicates excellent ovarian reserve; 6 to 9 is good; 9 to 10 is fair; 10 to 13 is diminished; and 13+ means that there may be very few good-quality eggs left in the ovaries. In terms of diminishing ovarian reserve or early menopause, FSH levels of about 10 to 12 mIU/ml may mean that you are starting to enter the beginning stages. Very high FSH levels (typically more than 30 mIU/ml) suggest that your ovarian function is significantly impaired.

As a woman ages, her FSH becomes elevated in an attempt to force the aging ovaries to respond. However, the exact mechanism responsible for this remains unknown. A rise in early-follicular-phase FSH is also accompanied by a decline in oocyte, or egg, quality, and some researchers have linked such FSH elevations with fetal abnormalities. In fact, it has been theorized that subtle but measurable increases in FSH precede the end of menstruation by approximately five years in some women.

In one fertility center, women undergoing in vitro fertilization (IVF) with a day 3 FSH of less than 15 mIU/ml were twice as likely to conceive as women with FSH values between 15 and 24.9 mIU/ml. Other investigators confirmed these results, and FSH values emerged as superior to maternal age as a method of determining reproductive outcome in IVF. Indeed, when day 3 FSH levels exceed 20 mIU/ml, conception rates fall sharply.

Because FSH levels fluctuate from month to month, it is likely that your FSH levels will vary, too. It is important to check your FSH levels several times over the course of a few months. Pay attention to any trends and how much above normal your FSH values usually remain. If you have several FSH levels on the "higher" end, it is likely that you are getting closer to ovarian insufficiency or the cessation of your menstrual cycle. At a minimum, you should have two FSH tests conducted at least a month apart.

ESTROGEN (ESTRADIOL)

FSH testing should always be accompanied by estrogen testing. Estradiol is the primary form of estrogen. When your ovaries begin to diminish and you start entering menopause, your estradiol levels decrease. In order to get an accurate diagnosis, it is critical to evaluate your estrogen levels to see if they are lower than normal. Normal estradiol levels on day 3 of your menstrual cycle should fall somewhere between 25 and 75 pg/ml. The higher your estradiol level is, the farther away from experiencing diminished ovarian function you probably are. Usually, high levels of estradiol can be an indication of other problems, such as cysts, so it is important to consider the big picture and never make assumptions based on a single hormone value.

ESTRADIOL LEVELS	
Nonmenopausal	**pg/ml**
Follicular phase	24–138
Luteal phase	19–164
Periovulatory	107–402
Postmenopausal	**pg/ml**
No hormone therapy	<36
With hormone therapy	18–361

Even if your estradiol level falls within the normal range, it can still be a sign of diminishing ovarian function when looked at with other hormones. The results of the different tests are interpreted together when making a diagnosis.

Irregular periods can be one sign of low estrogen levels. Low estrogen levels can also contribute to hampered fertility, hot flashes, insomnia, achy joints, headaches, moodiness, anxiety, changes in sexual desire, urinary tract infections, and bone loss. If you experience any of these symptoms, get your estrogen levels checked and consult your health care providers about possible treatment options to reduce the symptoms and possible other side effects.

Other Hormones

While you are at it, it is probably a good idea to have your other hormones evaluated, even if they aren't as important an indication of ovarian insufficiency. Hormones are complicated, and they often affect one another. If all your hormone levels are checked, this will provide you with more information about how to best proceed with a proper diagnosis and treatment plan.

Androgens are important for all women. The most common androgen tested for is testosterone. Throughout a woman's life, testosterone levels drop each year. However, for women with ovarian insufficiency, this decline in testosterone is much more sudden and can contribute to many of the menopause-related symptoms such as hot flashes and changes in sexual function. Normal total testosterone levels for a woman in her reproductive years are somewhere between 6 ng/dl and 86 ng/dl. However, anything above 50 ng/dl would be considered somewhat elevated. Elevated levels can suggest other problems with the ovaries or adrenal glands (very small hormone-secreting glands located at the tops of your kidneys). Measuring testosterone in women is fraught with difficulty. Most labs are using tests where the male levels are the standard. Since women have levels one tenth that of men, these tests are not very accurate at the low end of the spectrum.

Dehydroepiandrosterone sulfate (DHEAS) is another androgen that is not routinely measured in women. Abnormal DHEAS levels can be an indication of adrenal gland problems, which can inhibit your menstrual cycle and cause other reproduction-related problems. A normal DHEAS level is somewhere between 35 and 430 µg/dl, but different labs may have different "normals."

LH is another important hormone. As we saw earlier in this chapter, LH works in conjunction with FSH to stimulate ovulation. Overall, you want the amount of LH to roughly equal the amount of FSH to create a 1:1 ratio during the early part of your cycle as the egg begins to develop. If this is not the case, it could indicate problems. If your FSH level is higher, it suggests ovarian insufficiency. If your LH is higher, it could indicate polycystic ovary syndrome (PCOS), a hormone disorder that shares many of the same symptoms of ovarian insufficiency. Since LH also helps release the egg by surging—usually tripling in amount about 48 hours prior to ovulation—abnormal LH levels can inhibit your ability to ovulate, which will be a problem if you are interested in becoming pregnant.

Progesterone is another hormone that stimulates and regulates body functions. Most important, it plays a role in maintaining a pregnancy. Low levels of progesterone contribute to skipped periods and indicate a lack of ovulation. High levels of progesterone can cause symptoms such as PMS, breast tenderness, tiredness, feelings of being bloated, and mood swings. Progesterone levels vary widely during the menstrual cycle. But a "normal" level during day 3 should be less than 1.5 ng/ml.

The hormone prolactin should be considered as well. Prolactin is a hormone secreted by the pituitary gland, a pea-size gland located in your brain. Irregularities in your prolactin levels can inhibit ovulation and menstruation. Normal prolactin levels are less than 24 ng/ml. If your levels fall toward the high end of that spectrum or above, there is a good chance that you are experiencing problems with your pituitary gland.

Thyroid-simulating hormone (TSH) is tested to determine if the thyroid is functioning normally. A normal TSH level on day 3 is between 0.4 and 4 mIU/l. A midrange level in most labs is about 1.7. An abnormal TSH level (either too high or too low) can indicate thyroid disorders that may be affecting your periods and ovulation.

REPEAT TESTING

Because hormones fluctuate from day to day, month to month, it is important to have them checked a few times to document any changes or problems. Hormone levels can vary greatly, from normal to slightly out of range to very much out of range and back. Women who miss periods or have any menopause-related symptoms should have their hormones tested again in a few months. A diagnosis should *never* be given based on a single test at any specific time.

There's a Lot We Still Don't Know

Because women don't get their hormone levels checked routinely, there is still a lot we don't know about women's hormones and what levels are considered "normal." Most women get their hormones checked only when there is a problem. As a result, the data we have about hormones are primarily from women who experience some sort of hormonal or reproductive issue. As they relate to women without obvious hormone issues, we do not know as much as we would like about:

- Normal variations in the general population of women
- How variations in the hormone levels of women who have regular periods might have other subtle effects on their bodies and/or their sense of well-being
- What the normal progression of the hormone life cycle is

In reality, there might be many women experiencing some level of hormonal changes who do not experience the signs and symptoms of diminishing ovarian function. Unfortunately, not much research has been conducted on this topic. The good news is that this is changing and there are researchers who are dedicating their professional careers to this area.

We need to understand how hormones usually decline over a woman's lifetime and how this relates to women who experience menstrual disruptions or insufficient ovarian function. In order to determine this, we need to have more women testing their hormones and more researchers analyzing these data. By building a larger database, we will be able to better determine what exactly is "normal," or at least "typical." Only then can we begin learning how to discern exactly what is causing problems and come up with new methods and treatments for preventing any further problems.

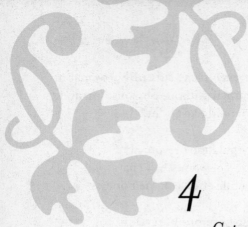

4

Get a Diagnosis

*If I hadn't been diagnosed with POI, I never would have known how
lucky some people are to be able to conceive naturally, how strong
some people are to battle with infertility for so long, an appreciation
for people whose health problems are worse, the support and
friendship that I have, how wise some people are, how fantastic my
husband is, how strong and driven I can be, how insensitive other
people can be when they don't understand, the use of chocolate
to give you a boost, and how my reproductive system should
(and does) work.*

—Valerie

THERE IS NO WAY to describe typical menstrual or ovarian activity
changes among women with ovarian insufficiency. For some women,
symptoms start virtually overnight. They are fine one day and start experiencing all sorts of symptoms the next. For others, symptoms start
gradually—a missed period or feeling mildly flushed. Often they assume they are pregnant, only to receive a negative pregnancy test. In any
case, all too often they are left wondering what is happening to their
bodies.

Because many doctors are finally beginning to recognize the signs
and symptoms of ovarian insufficiency in younger women, more
women are being properly diagnosed. The symptoms of decreasing
ovarian function can be similar to those of going through "natural,"
more age-appropriate menopause, but the emotions and overall experi-

ence are not. Women who experience menopause-related symptoms at a much younger age commonly report a wide variety of experiences, including the following.

Irregular Periods

As we said earlier (and as you've probably experienced yourself), irregular periods are often the first and most prominent sign that something might be amiss with your body. Irregular periods start occurring in the early stages of diminishing ovarian function. Periods become unpredictable, sometimes coming sooner than twenty-eight days or much later than you are used to. You may begin to have lighter-than-usual or heavier-than-usual periods lasting for a short amount of time or lingering for what seems like forever. You may even start to skip a month here or there, then have a few normal months, only to skip again. Overall inconsistency becomes the norm.

What does this all mean? When your period comes more frequently (or less than every twenty-eight days), it may indicate that your hormones may be off kilter, causing your follicles to develop faster and resulting in a shorter cycle. Extremely light periods may mean you are not making enough hormones to build up your uterine lining or may be a sign that you are not ovulating. Very heavy bleeding may be another side of not ovulating, in addition to having an extra-thick uterine lining. Skipped periods may suggest that your ovarian function is declining. Declining ovarian function does permit your eggs to mature or for your uterine lining to thicken properly for pregnancy. Eventually, as ovarian function ceases altogether or menopause gets closer, your periods will stop altogether.

Unfortunately, many doctors don't realize the importance of good menstrual health and how irregular periods can be a sign that something else is going on. Often, a woman is told that her body will just work itself out on its own, or she will be prescribed birth control pills in order to regulate her periods. This will not cure ovarian insufficiency or delay diminishing ovarian function. Instead, it will only mask the symptoms as problems continue to progress.

Irregular periods almost always signal that something is happening within your body that is affecting your hormones. About 10 to 28 percent of those with primary amenorrhea (meaning women who have not

gotten a first period by age sixteen) are diagnosed with ovarian insufficiency. About 4 to 18 percent with secondary amenorrhea (meaning
that they had periods—perhaps even regular cycles—that have stopped
for at least three months) have some form of ovarian insufficiency.

If you experience periods that regularly come more than thirty-five
days apart, or if you go more than three months without a period, it is
important that you talk with your doctor. Don't accept "It's no big deal"
or "Don't worry about it" for an answer. Something is going on, and it is
up to you to be proactive in finding out what this something is so you
can effectively deal with it.

Other Reproductive Changes

For women with more age-appropriate menopause, this time marks an
end of childbearing potential and often a sense of relief from decades of
menstruation-related issues. But for women who experience diminishing ovarian function and are in the midst of their prime childbearing
years, menopause takes on an entirely different meaning. It can signal
an abrupt end to the ability to have children, sometimes before childbearing has even begun. Reproductive changes are typically the most
noticeable and dramatic physical changes affecting women.

INFERTILITY

Many women do not fully notice the changes, particularly the irregular
periods, until they start trying to become pregnant. Even if you are
still having periods, your cycle might not work well enough to conceive
or sustain a pregnancy. Often this is a double blow—learning that your
ovarian function is diminishing *and* you might be unable to become
pregnant on your own.

LOW LIBIDO

Many things influence our sex drive: psychology, environment, circum-
stance, and of course hormones. Any way you slice it, hormones play a
role in our feelings toward sex. Because ovarian insufficiency impacts
hormones, it is no surprise that sometimes libido suffers. However, it
seems that some women are more prone to these effects than others.

Usually, the worse your other symptoms, the more your sex drive will be affected. Still, when you are young, any negative impact on your sexuality can be distressing. Remember that while hormone shifts account for some of your sexual experiences, life circumstances, expectations, and other factors are big players as well. In fact, your brain is actually the most important sex organ.

Physical Changes

Diminishing ovarian function can lead to some very real physical symptoms. Most women will experience at least some of these symptoms, no matter what their age. They can last for years, as hormone levels fall and fluctuate. The severity of the symptoms often depends on how gradual or sudden the changes are.

BREAST TENDERNESS

This is a confusing one. Breast tenderness refers to swelling and feelings of tenderness, which can last a few days or even weeks. Most women who experience a diminution of ovarian function do not expect their symptoms to be related to it. More logical guesses as to the causes of breast tenderness are PMS or pregnancy. But with erratic hormones, the tenderness doesn't disappear with your periods or with pregnancy.

VAGINAL DRYNESS

When your estrogen levels drop, the vagina can become drier and less elastic. Additionally, your vagina can change shape, becoming shorter and tighter. As a result, sex might become more painful, or at the very least uncomfortable. You may also become more prone to vaginal infections or experience more irritation.

HOT FLASHES

Hot flashes (also known as hot flushes) and menopause seem to go hand in hand. This is menopause's trademark symptom and is caused by blood vessels expanding, which makes more blood flow to the skin. Most women going through diminishing ovarian function (regardless of age and cause) experience hot flashes at some point. For younger women, this experience can be more intense. The quicker your estrogen levels drop, the more likely you will produce more hot flashes. Hot flashes can vary in intensity from just needing a little fanning now and again to feeling as if you just stepped into a fire.

Usually, hot flashes start with a prickly feeling down your back, indicating that something strange is coming on. As your internal temperature drops abruptly, your skin begins to heat up (literally, sometimes by a few degrees), extending toward your back, chest, neck, face, and scalp. If you touch your skin, it may feel as if you have been sitting out in the sun for hours. Hot flashes can last for a few seconds to several minutes.

NIGHT SWEATS

Night sweats are similar to hot flashes, but they occur at night. In response to the rise in your core temperature, your skin sweats, giving off heat and trying to balance itself. You then get all hot and sweaty. Finally, as your sweat begins to evaporate, you get so chilled that you struggle to get warm again. These extreme sensations can jolt you awake and constantly interrupt your sleep.

INSOMNIA/DISRUPTED SLEEP

Sleep may also be disrupted in other ways. If you have always had a difficult time sleeping, this can be exacerbated. You might find your sleep is less restful than before, or you might have difficulty getting any sleep at all. This lack of sleep, mixed with out-of-whack hormones, can lead to daytime fatigue or lack of energy.

BLADDER CONTROL PROBLEMS

As mentioned above, hormonal changes can lead to less elastic vaginal muscles. The same can be said for all the muscles in your pelvic region, including those that control your bladder. Lower levels of estrogen often contribute to less elastic muscles throughout that area. While you may notice that you have to urinate more often or with more urgency, most women find this symptom more annoying than life altering.

PALPITATIONS

Heart palpitations can be frightening no matter why they happen. Palpitations are when your heart suddenly starts pounding faster and faster until it feels as if it's going to explode out of your chest. It can happen to anyone at any time, even if you are sitting calmly or relaxing. For some reason, palpitations seem to be more prevalent among women going through hormonal changes and often accompany hot flashes.

HEADACHES

There is a connection between hormones and headaches. Many women experience headaches whenever their hormones fluctuate. As estrogen levels drop or progesterone levels increase, headaches tend to get worse. They can range from frequent annoying headaches to full-blown migraines. When hormones start to subside, most headaches go away.

GASTROINTESTINAL DISTRESS

Since so many changes are happening to your body, it is not uncommon to experience more gas, indigestion, heartburn, or nausea. Feeling bloated is a common complaint, too, although it is uncertain how it relates to hormone changes.

JOINT OR MUSCLE SORENESS

Estrogen deficiency can sometimes lead to an all-over achy feeling affecting your joints and major muscles. Sometimes this is misdiagnosed as the flu, fibromyalgia, or chronic fatigue syndrome.

DIZZINESS OR LIGHT-HEADEDNESS

This can occur in conjunction with hot flashes or on its own. Many women experiencing hormonal changes complain of periodic feelings of dizziness or light-headedness.

DRY MOUTH AND SENSITIVE GUMS

Believe it or not, oral health is associated with hormones. Your mouth may become unusually dry, or you may have difficulty brushing your teeth due to sensitive gums. In either case, don't be surprised if your mouth starts to feel the effects of hormonal changes.

INCREASED ALLERGIES

Many types of allergies are a result of hormone reactions. In fact, allergies become more prevalent as normal hormonal functions change. Types of allergies associated with hormonal changes include hay fever, asthma, itchy eyes, eczema, and hives.

Changes in Appearance

When menopause and natural aging are synonymous, many of the changes in appearance are accepted or embraced. Ideally, women proudly come "into their age." Younger women do not have the same feelings when they begin to experience a decrease in ovarian function. Changing hormones and their impact on overall appearance make women feel much older than they really are. In a culture where youth is desirable and women strive to stay young-looking, this can be a devastating experience.

WEIGHT GAIN

Gaining weight around your waist or abdomen is often referred to as "male-pattern" weight gain. This "apple" shape is more common among men. "Female-pattern" weight gain often results in a more "pear" shape, with extra weight settling around the hips, thighs, and buttocks. After ovarian function begins to diminish, women's metabolisms change and fat tends to be redistributed even when they keep up their diet and exercise routines. Maintain a healthy weight in order to help prevent cardiovascular disease or other long-term health concerns. Talk with your health care provider or nutritionist about any concerns you have about your weight and how to best go about losing weight.

DRY OR ITCHY SKIN

Dryness seems to be a common theme during hormonal changes. Also, your skin may feel supersensitive or tingle.

WRINKLES

While some wrinkling is due to aging, additional hormonal changes cause skin to lose some of its elasticity and become thinner. Wrinkles may start to appear in the delicate tissues around the eyes, cheeks, and lips. These can result in "crow's feet" or smile lines in areas that were once smooth and supple.

HAIR LOSS OR THINNING

Because hair follicles need estrogen, hair loss or thinning among women is a result of lower levels of estrogen. Hair coming out as you brush it or unusually dry or brittle hair can be an initial sign of changing hormones.

INCREASED FACIAL HAIR

Given the low levels of female hormones in your body, your male hormones have a great influence on increased facial hair growth. This can include increased hair (or darker, coarser hair) on the chin, upper lip, chest (including around your nipples), or abdomen.

CHANGES IN BODY ODOR

Increased body odor associated with hormone changes doesn't have anything to do with perspiration. Normal bacteria are having a heyday because your metabolism is changing and your body is ridding itself of excess waste due to hormonal imbalances. Body odor can present as foot odor, sweaty or smelly hands, bad breath, or armpit odor.

CHANGES IN NAILS

As hormones fluctuate, fingernails and toenails can become softer and crack or break more easily.

DRY EYES

Because changes in hormones typically contribute to the drying out of the skin, why not the eyes, too? These types of hormonal changes make women more likely to experience dry eyes and accompanying symptoms such as eye irritation and blurred vision.

Emotional Changes

Changing hormone levels (whatever the cause) can create an emotional roller coaster. Often, these symptoms are more prominent than the more physical symptoms. With ovarian insufficiency, unlike in more traditional menopause, this is not a time to celebrate or to look forward to that "postmenopausal zest"—what Margaret Mead originally described as a wave of relief, knowing that you have survived the perimenopausal chaos. The emotional toll that diminishing ovarian function takes, in addition to the typical emotional changes initiated by changing hormone levels, can lead to an even more harrowing emotional experience.

FOGGY FEELINGS

Sometimes changing hormone levels cause women to feel "not quite right." This may include an overall "fogginess" or feelings of general malaise. Unfortunately, it is difficult to pinpoint the exact feelings other than that something odd is going on.

IRRITABILITY AND AGGRESSIVENESS

If you are feeling irritable or unusually aggressive, there is a good chance it is connected to your changing hormones. In fact, this is one of the most common emotional changes that women experience.

MOOD SWINGS

Mood swings are another major emotional change sparked by changing hormone levels. Some women liken these changes to PMS—only constant. Reacting to changing levels of estrogen, women experience highs, lows, and everything in between. Though feelings of sadness or "blues" are typical as ovarian function diminishes, severe or clinical depression is not a symptom and should be further evaluated if experienced.

NERVOUSNESS AND ANXIETY

With anxiety, there is a sense of foreboding or that something is terribly wrong. Anxiety-related symptoms include trembling, sweating, and being easily startled.

MEMORY LAPSES

Memory problems may also be related to ovarian insufficiency. Even though there are no known connections between memory and changing hormones, many women experience some sort of short-term memory loss. Some believe that this is related to the stress associated with going though ovarian insufficiency, especially when it occurs at a young age.

CONFUSION OR LACK OF CONCENTRATION

Women experiencing hormone changes may also have difficulty concentrating. It is important to keep your mind engaged and stimulated in order to lessen the effects of this symptom.

FATIGUE AND LACK OF ENERGY

Fatigue is one of the most common symptoms of hormone fluctuations. It is described as an ongoing and persistent feeling of weakness, tiredness, and lowered energy level. While many women also experience difficulty sleeping, fatigue is more lack of energy than drowsiness. While fatigue and lack of energy are not emotional symptoms per se, these symptoms can easily exacerbate many other emotional symptoms you may be feeling.

Testing for Ovarian Insufficiency

It is important to note that all of these symptoms can be an indication of something else going on with your body besides ovarian insufficiency or early menopause. If you experience any of these symptoms, it is important to discuss them with your doctor. Because some doctors are slow to consider ovarian insufficiency or early menopause as a cause, it is also critical to keep asking questions until you are satisfied. Sometimes this may mean finding a new health care provider with more experience in the areas of ovarian insufficiency and early menopause. All of these symptoms are very real, so never settle for the old "Don't worry, it's all in your head" routine.

Unfortunately, there is not one definitive test for ovarian insufficiency or early menopause. Therefore, be prepared for a wide range of testing. You and your doctor will have to sit down together and discuss the results of all your tests in order to get an accurate picture.

PHYSICAL EXAM

Most young women neglect getting a routine physical exam by their primary care provider. Even if you are feeling healthy, it is important to get a checkup, including your whole body, not just any gynecological concerns. Besides finding and treating any health problems early, routine exams also help you develop an ongoing relationship with your health care provider. This way, he or she can better determine your specific risks and vulnerabilities as you grow older. If you are in your twenties or thirties, it is important to get a full physical exam about every two to three years. For women in their forties, it should be done every year or two.

Exams should start with your filling out your medical history questionnaire as thoroughly and thoughtfully as possible. Include any family history of any type of medical problem, physical or mental—even if you don't think it is important. Come prepared with your own list of concerns and questions to discuss with your doctor. Don't leave anything out, and don't leave until all your questions have been answered to your satisfaction.

During each exam, your doctor should look at your skin, listen to your heart and lungs, feel your abdominal area, look at your eyes, and take your blood pressure. Also, a comprehensive blood analysis should be conducted to check for sugar, cholesterol, liver and kidney function, and other indicators. As discussed in the previous chapter, hormones should be assessed if you are experiencing any changes with your menstrual cycle or if you are concerned about your fertility. This will help you and your health care provider identify any problems as soon as possible. Discuss all your menopause-related symptoms, since additional tests might be needed.

MENSTRUAL HISTORY

Most women are fairly consistent about getting regular gynecological care. For women over the age of twenty-one and younger women who are sexually active, it is good to get a gynecological exam every year. During these visits, your health care provider will give you an internal exam, do a Pap test (to check for cervical cancer), check for sexually transmitted infections, and do a breast exam. If you are over forty, a mammogram will also be suggested.

Of course, there is that routine question: "When was the first day of your last period?" Many women do not dwell too long on this topic and respond quickly and simply.

However, this is a good time to stop and think about your menstrual history:

- Has anything changed lately?
- Are your periods coming more often or less often?
- Have you been having any breakthrough bleeding (bleeding between periods)?
- Have your periods become longer or shorter?
- Are they more painful?
- Are you experiencing any other new or strange symptoms related to your cycle?

All these issues can indicate other problems, including ovarian insufficiency or early menopause. At the end of the book, there is a chart you can use to track your menstrual cycles and related symptoms.

FAMILY HISTORY

It is important for your provider to understand where you are coming from, in terms of your family medical history.

- Did anyone in your family (especially close family members such as sisters, aunts, or your mother) experience infertility?

- Has anyone in your family been diagnosed with any type of chronic disease, such as an auto-immune disorder or genetic condition?
- At what age did your mother, aunts, and grandmothers go through menopause or start to experience menstrual irregularities?

Again, these answers can provide an insight into what you can expect. In fact, the biggest predictor of when you will experience menopause is when your mother went through menopause. If she experienced it early, you are likely to do so as well.

Because most young women do not have a regular doctor and seek care with a variety of health care providers, you are going to have to get used to repeating a lot of this information. It's up to you to be on top of things and remain proactive. Some women find it easiest to write everything down and carry the list with them to their doctors' visits. The most powerful diagnostic tool you have is sharing information about your medical history. If you aren't satisfied with the answers your health care provider gives you, don't just ignore a problem. Find someone else who will answer all your questions and will work with you to find a solution.

PART TWO

Why Me?

It's More Common

than You Think

5

Health-Related Causes
of Early Menopause

IN SOME CASES, THE cause of your symptoms is obvious: your ovaries
have been surgically removed, you have undergone intensive treatments
for cancer, or you have a clear family history of ovarian insufficiency.
Still, in almost 90 percent of cases, the exact cause is unknown. However, many doctors and researchers are learning more and more about
what may contribute to diminished ovarian function and early menopause. Let's look at some of these causes. If you have a history of any of
these diseases or disorders, it's important for you to discuss it with your
doctor to see if it could be a underlying cause of your ovarian insufficiency symptoms.

Autoimmune Disorders

One category of disorders that may contribute to diminishing ovarian
function is autoimmune disorders. Some researchers estimate that
nearly a third of women with ovarian insufficiency have signs of an autoimmune disorder. Autoimmune disturbances may begin before ovarian dysfunction becomes apparent. In general, autoimmune disorders
are caused by an overactive immune response by the body in which the

body begins to attack itself. Hormone levels have been shown to affect the severity of some autoimmune diseases. As a result, the reproductive organs, including the ovaries, are sometimes major targets of an autoimmune attack.

Still, it becomes sort of a chicken-and-egg conundrum. Do immune diseases and disorders cause ovarian insufficiency, or does ovarian insufficiency lead to a higher risk of developing certain conditions?

We all need a healthy immune system to fight off invaders, such as bacteria and viruses. They can kill us, so our body needs to recognize them and destroy them. Because our bodies are made of the same building blocks as viruses and bacteria, it is no surprise that now and then the immune system makes a mistake and attacks something that is "self." One example is rheumatoid arthritis. Some people with this condition get swollen, red joints that deform the fingers. That's the immune system recognizing something in the joint that's foreign and attacking it. The same thing can happen in the glands that control hormones.

WHEN THE OVARY IS ATTACKED

"Some women have an autoimmune attack against the ovary," explains Dr. Lawrence Nelson, "but some women have an autoimmune attack not against the entire ovary but against these follicles that are trying to grow. In that situation, if we could recognize who those patients are, as a cause of ovarian failure, and have a treatment to suppress the immune system, we might be able to get those follicles to work just long enough for a pregnancy to occur."

He continues, "The major problem about autoimmune ovarian failure is that there is no accurate blood test to tell us who has it. We have accurate blood tests for rheumatoid arthritis. We have accurate blood tests for autoimmune diseases of the thyroid, but there is not an accurate blood test to tell us who has an autoimmune attack against the ovary, and that's been a major obstacle to making a diagnosis."

THYROID FUNCTION

Women with insufficient ovaries also tend to have issues with their thyroid gland. Often, this involves having low thyroid function, or hypothyroidism. The thyroid controls the body's metabolism and energy levels, so a low level of thyroid hormone can affect a woman's metabolism and result in low energy levels. Symptoms of a thyroid problem can include mental and physical sluggishness as well as cold feet. A recent study showed that about 30 percent of women with POI/POF also had low thyroid function, compared to only 2 percent in the general population.

ADDISON'S DISEASE

Addison's disease is an autoimmune disorder that attacks the adrenal glands, which are part of the endocrine system located just above the kidneys. The adrenal glands produce hormones that regulate the body's response to stress and its handling of salt. Recent studies have shown that more than 3 percent of women with POI also have Addison's disease.

Symptoms of Addison's disease include loss of appetite, weight loss, dizziness, and fatigue. The most effective way to test for Addison's disease is to conduct an adrenal antibody test as well as an ACTH stimulation test through blood samples. While there is no way to prevent Addison's disease, it can be easily managed by taking medications. If left untreated, Addison's disease can be life-threatening, because the body cannot respond properly to stressful events, such as severe illness, injury, or surgery.

LUPUS

Lupus is an autoimmune disease that affects the joints and internal organs. The most common complaints of those who have lupus are fatigue, loss of appetite, muscle pain, arthritis, rash, photosensitivity, and mouth and nose ulcerations. Lupus and ovarian insufficiency also have some common symptoms, including sleep problems, heart palpitations, headaches and hot flashes, weight gain, mood swings, and irregular periods. Either the disease itself or the medications that are used to treat it can cause women to experience diminishing ovarian function.

TYPE 1 DIABETES

Women with type 1 diabetes (also known as insulin-dependent diabetes mellitus, or IDDM) often experience a greater prevalence of menstrual disorders than do women without diabetes. Still, there is very little research looking at these women's experiences with menopause to indicate whether menopause timing is affected. The Familial Autoimmune and Diabetes (FAD) Study showed that more than 30 percent of women with type 1 diabetes experienced several risk factors often associated with ovarian insufficiency, including menstrual irregularities before age thirty, not having children, and the removal of one ovary. This rate is more than double that found among the general nondiabetic population of women. One explanation for this may be related to prolonged hyperglycemia and/or other long-term complications of diabetes. Genetics may be another reason for the relationship between diabetes and ovarian insufficiency. Genetic factors that increase diabetes risk may also increase the risk of autoimmune disorders and influence the age of menopause.

POLYGLANDULAR DEFICIENCY SYNDROMES

Polyglandular deficiency syndromes involve several poorly functioning endocrine glands and are autoimmune in nature. Because everyone experiences these syndromes differently, it often takes years of observation and testing before a diagnosis is given. Type I polyglandular failure occurs in early childhood (typically between the ages of three and five) or in adulthood before age twenty-five. Type I polyglandular failure most often includes problems such as hypoparathyroidism and andrenocortical failure and can also affect the development of reproductive organs in children. Type II (also known as Schmidt's syndrome) occurs in adults around the age of thirty, most commonly among women, and involves the adrenal grand, thyroid gland, and pancreas, resulting in type 1 diabetes.

HYPOPARATHYROIDISM

Hypoparathyroidism is the decreased function of the parathyroid gland, which is located in your throat just below your voice box and near your thyroid gland. This condition is extremely rare and typically occurs because of some type of damage or removal of these glands during surgery. Overall, when the parathyroid gland is not functioning adequately, it leads to decreased levels of calcium and increased levels of phosphorus in the blood. In addition to diminished ovarian function, symptoms range from mild tingling in the hands and fingers and around the mouth to severe forms of muscle cramps affecting the entire body.

FIBROMYALGIA SYNDROME

Some doctors think a connection exists between fibromyalgia and diminished ovarian function. Fibromyalgia syndrome involves pain in the muscle, and connective tissue. Other features are fatigue, sleep disturbance, and joint stiffness. Fibromyalgia also contributes to menopause-related symptoms such as anxiety, depression, joint pain, gastrointestinal problems, and hot flashes. According to research published in the February 2009 issue of *Clinical Rheumatology*, women with fibromyalgia were most likely to have diminishing ovarian function or to have had a hysterectomy. Additionally, they often reported experiencing more severe menopause-type symptoms. Researchers believe there is some sort of hormonal link to fibromyalgia that explains why women are much more likely than men to develop the disease.

OTHER AUTOIMMUNE DISORDERS

A few other common autoimmune disorders, including chronic fatigue syndrome (CFS), irritable bowel syndrome (IBS), and rheumatoid arthritis (RA) may be linked to ovarian insufficiency as well. Myasthenia gravis may also be related to ovarian deficiency; it is a chronic autoimmune neuromuscular disease characterized by varying degrees of muscle weakness. Unfortunately, little research has been conducted to determine the true relationship; however, patients' experiences and anecdotal evidence suggest there might be a connection. If you have any of these diseases, it is important to discuss them with your doctor to better understand how they are impacting your ovarian function.

Genetic Diseases

After autoimmune disorders, genetics is the next most frequently identified cause of ovarian insufficiency. Genetic diseases are passed along through the genes from parent to child. A genetic disorder is a disease caused by abnormalities in an individual's genetic material (genome). A karyotype is recommended for POI patients less than thirty years old to exclude hereditary risks. A karyotype is a test used to check for chromosome abnormalities. It creates a picture of all the chromosomes from an individual's cells. A simple blood sample provides enough information for the testing. A picture of a person's chromosomes is created by staining the chromosomes with a special dye, photographing them through a microscope, and arranging them in pairs. The karyotype gives information about the number of chromosomes a person has, the structure of the chromosomes, and the sex of the individual.

Some common chromosomal or genetic diseases that may contribute to ovarian insufficiency include:

- **Galactosemia.** This is a rare genetic metabolic disorder. People who have galactosemia lack a liver enzyme needed to digest foods with lactose, such as milk, cheese, and butter. If left untreated, as many as 75 percent of babies born with galactosemia will die. While many girls and women with galactosemia experience primary ovarian insufficiency, the exact relationship is unclear.
- **Fragile X.** This is the most common inherited form of intellectual disabilities. One in 130 women is estimated to be a carrier of the fragile X mutation. Having this FMR1 gene affected can also cause women to develop fragile X–associated primary ovarian insufficiency (or FXPOI). Since fragile X carriers often do not exhibit any outward symptoms, irregular menstrual cycles may be the only indication that they are at risk. A DNA test can determine if an individual is a fragile X carrier.
- **Turner syndrome.** This is a genetic condition in which a female does not have the usual pair of two X chromosomes. Turner syndrome occurs in about 1 out of every 2,000 live births. Usually diagnosed in infants (or even before birth), early symptoms include swollen hands and feet and wide and webbed necks. As these girls age, additional symptoms become apparent, such as absent or in-

complete development at puberty (including sparse pubic hair and small breasts); a broad, flat chest shaped like a shield; drooping eyelids; dry eyes; and short height. Also, nearly 90 percent of those with Turner syndrome will experience ovarian insufficiency leading to vaginal dryness, painful intercourse, absent menstruation, and infertility.

- **Thalassemia.** This is an inherited blood disorder seen most frequently in people from Mediterranean countries, North Africa, the Middle East, India, Central Asia, and Southeast Asia. Thalassemia causes the body to make fewer healthy red blood cells and less hemoglobin than normal. For women with thalassemia, major iron overload in the blood may contribute to developing ovarian insufficiency.

- **Primary hemochromatosis.** One of the most common inherited diseases (about 0.5 percent of the U.S. Caucasian population carries the genetic defect that makes them susceptible to the disease), hemochromatosis leads to severe iron overload. The extra iron builds up in the body's organs and damages them. For women, it can cause ovarian dysfunction even before symptoms begin to develop and the disease is diagnosed.

- **Androgen insensitivity syndrome (AIS).** This is also referred to as androgen resistance syndrome and occurs in up to 1 in 20,000 people. People with this condition are genetically male, with one X chromosome and one Y chromosome in each cell. Because their bodies are unable to respond to certain male sex hormones (called androgens), they may have mostly female sex characteristics or signs of both male and female sexual development. Those with female external sex characteristics do not have a uterus, are unable to menstruate, and will also experience infertility.

Family History

Women can learn a lot about what to expect with their reproductive cycles by talking with their female relatives.

AFFECTED FEMALE RELATIVE

Women with a family history of ovulation problems or early menopause are at higher risk for developing ovarian insufficiency. Women with one or more first-degree relatives (meaning a mother or sister) who experience the signs and symptoms of ovarian insufficiency at an early age are likely to experience the same. Since there is a variety of genetic factors in play, it is nearly impossible to accurately predict the exact age when ovarian function will start to decrease. However, a strong influence of heritability of ovarian insufficiency must be taken into account.

Because hormonal changes that lower ovarian function and fertility begin several years before outward signs of ovarian insufficiency become evident, women may not realize they are affected. Smart women make themselves aware of their own family's fertility history and the ages at which female relatives started to experience menopause-related symptoms. Don't be afraid to discuss these issues with members of your family. Not only is this important for having children, but premature changes in ovarian function can lead to depression, reduced libido, and increased risk for early onset of osteoporosis, heart disease, and Alzheimer's disease.

Viral Infections

Viral infections might also be related to developing ovarian insufficiency. If your mother suffered from a viral infection while she was pregnant, this could affect your ovarian development. Likewise, if you have suffered from a viral infection such as mumps, the infection could have spread to your ovaries, interfering with their function. As a result, you might either produce fewer eggs than most women or run out of eggs more quickly.

Other Causes

Because all aspects of ovarian insufficiency are severely underresearched, we don't know a lot about what exactly causes diminishing ovarian function in some women. One example, idiopathic thrombocytopenic purpura (ITP), also known as Werlhof's disease, is the condition of having a low platelet count with no known cause (commonly referred to as idiopathic). There are about 50 to 100 new cases of ITP per million each year, including both children and adults. For adults, the condition is chronic and affects more women than men. Symptoms of ITP include the development of bruises or red spots under the skin, nosebleeds, and bleeding at the gums.

UNEXPLAINED OVARIAN INSUFFICIENCY

For the vast majority of women who experience ovarian insufficiency, the cause remains unknown. However, because ovarian insufficiency is associated with a wide range of other serious conditions, it is important to rule out the other diseases first. And just because it seems unexplained now does not mean that links with other diseases won't be found later. In addition, appropriate treatment depends on understanding what is going on with your body as much as possible.

6

Ovarian Insufficiency
Due to Surgery

At thirty-eight, I had a hysterectomy. I went on a tailspin straight into menopause. No one told me about the shock my body would be going through. I am forty-two now and am just now starting to feel back on track.

—Susanna

A HYSTERECTOMY IS A medical procedure; it generally refers to any operation to remove a woman's reproductive organs. However, there are many variations on a hysterectomy, depending on which reproductive organs are removed. More accurately, a *hysterectomy* involves the uterus, while an *oophorectomy,* which often accompanies a hysterectomy, involves the ovaries. In either case, hysterectomy and menopause are two words that often go together, because when the uterus is removed, whether or not the ovaries remain, a woman will stop having periods. However, hysterectomies are not just limited to women in their later years. Many younger women are faced with the decision whether to have a hysterectomy or not. How does this experience affect them? And how can they best cope?

Reasons for a Hysterectomy

A hysterectomy may be recommended because a woman's life is negatively impacted by issues related to her reproductive organs or menstrual cycle. There are several good reasons to have a hysterectomy, including:

- To save your life, usually when cancer, severe bleeding, or infection is involved
- To correct severe prolapse, when the uterus falls out of place and causes obstructions
- To relieve pain—you may be experiencing significant pain and bleeding that affect your daily function and ability to live life fully

Even in these cases, a hysterectomy should be done only as a last resort, when no other less drastic measures are available.

Sometimes a hysterectomy is done before a clear diagnosis is achieved. In the past, a hysterectomy was performed to relieve symptoms, not treat a disease. While the goal is to stop symptoms such as bleeding and pain, it is important to know the cause of the symptoms before a hysterectomy is performed. For younger women, the removal of the reproductive organs may result in additional symptoms related to the absence of the organs and the accompanying lower hormone levels. Before scheduling any type of surgery, it is important for a woman to look into the details of her diagnosis and understand why a hysterectomy is being suggested. Always ask questions, particularly about alternative and less invasive solutions. And second opinions can help greatly. There might be other, equally effective methods for treating certain symptoms, such as bleeding. Every woman and every situation is different.

A good treatment option for one woman might not be ideal for another. The table below indicates some potential alternatives to hysterectomies that you can discuss with your health care provider. Getting a second opinion is always wise before undergoing any type of surgery.

ALTERNATIVES TO HYSTERECTOMY

Drug therapy	Certain medications may lessen the symptoms, such as heavy bleeding or pain.
Endometrial ablation	With a special device, your doctor uses electricity, heat, or cold to destroy the uterine lining and stop bleeding.
Uterine artery embolization	This procedure is used to treat fibroids and involves blocking the blood supply to the tumors. Over time, the fibroids shrink.
Myomectomy	This surgical procedure removes a portion of the uterus but leaves the rest of the uterus intact.
Vaginal pessary	In this procedure, an object is inserted into the vagina to hold the womb in place. Vaginal pessaries come in many shapes and sizes, so they must be fitted for each woman individually. They can be used temporarily or as a permanent form of treatment.
Endometrial resection	Similarly to endometrial ablation, the uterine lining is destroyed using an electrosurgical wire loop.

Hysterectomies are recommended for a variety of reasons. They are broken down statistically in the table below.

KEY CAUSES OF HYSTERECTOMY

Cause	Percent
Fibroids	30
Endometriosis	20
Uterine prolapse	16
Cancer	10
Dysfunctional uterine bleeding	Unknown
Chronic pelvic pain	Unknown
Other reasons (bleeding, infection, uterine rupture or inversion)	Unknown

Types of Hysterectomies

There are a number of types of hysterectomies. A hysterectomy is a surgical procedure usually done under general anesthesia. It can be performed through an abdominal incision or through the vagina. Sometimes these choices are not available to all patients due to various medical reasons, weight, diagnosis, size of the uterus, expertise of your surgeon, and other factors. Discuss your options with your surgeon, and always consider getting a second opinion from another surgeon. One surgeon may tell you that you are not a candidate for a less invasive procedure, but another may find you are an excellent candidate. Do your research!

TOTAL ABDOMINAL HYSTERECTOMY

A total abdominal hysterectomy is the most common type of hysterectomy. About 75 percent of all hysterectomies performed in the United States are total abdominal hysterectomies. During this procedure, your entire uterus, including the cervix, is removed through either a horizontal or vertical incision in the abdomen. Cancer of the ovary and uterus, endometriosis, and large uterine fibroids are commonly treated by a total abdominal hysterectomy. And although the ovaries may not be removed, many women still experience menopausal symptoms sooner than they would have otherwise.

VAGINAL HYSTERECTOMY

During this procedure, the uterus is removed directly through the vagina. The vagina is stretched and kept open by special instruments so no external incision is made, resulting in no scarring, a shorter hospital stay, and a quicker recovery time. A vaginal hysterectomy is most appropriate for uterine prolapse, endometrial hyperplasia, or cervical dysplasia. Overall, this type of hysterectomy is sometimes linked to higher rates of complications. This method can also affect sexual function because the vagina may be shortened or tightened during surgery, leading to uncomfortable intercourse.

LAPAROSCOPY-ASSISTED VAGINAL HYSTERECTOMY

Very similar to the vaginal hysterectomy, this procedure utilizes a laparoscope, a very thin viewing tube with a magnifying glass–like device at the end. Laparoscopy-assisted vaginal hysterectomy is sometimes preferred because it allows the upper abdomen to be carefully evaluated during surgery. This procedure is typically used for endometrial cancer or in conjunction with removal of the ovaries.

SUPRACERVICAL HYSTERECTOMY

A supracervical hysterectomy is used to remove the uterus while sparing the cervix, which is located at the very bottom of the uterus. When this is done, it leaves the cervix as a sort of "stump" for women who have no reason to have their cervix removed. Leaving the cervix intact allows added support of the vagina and may decrease the risk of vaginal prolapse. Women who are not good candidates for this type of procedure include women who have had abnormal Pap tests or are at high risk of developing cervical cancer. This is a slightly simpler procedure and can be performed more quickly than a total abdominal hysterectomy.

RADICAL HYSTERECTOMY

Because it involves removing both the uterus and upper vagina, a radical hysterectomy is rare and is considered very extensive surgery. This procedure is most commonly recommended for women suffering from cervical cancer in which pelvic lymph nodes might also be removed. There are more complications with this than with a simple abdominal hysterectomy, including possible injury to the bowels and urinary tract.

OOPHORECTOMY AND SALPINGO-OOPHORECTOMY

An oophorectomy is the surgical removal of the ovaries, while a salpingo-oophorectomy is the removal of the ovaries and the adjacent fallopian tubes. Both of these procedures are typically recommended in cases of cancer of the ovary or ovarian tumors. In these cases, oophorectomy and salpingo-oophorectomy normally accompanies a hysterectomy, which also removes the uterus.

These procedures can involve the removal of only one ovary or both, called a bilateral oophorectomy. The ovaries may also be removed due to ectopic pregnancy, endometriosis, benign or malignant tumors, ovarian cysts, and pelvic inflammatory disease. If only one ovary is removed, many women maintain normal hormone levels and sometimes may even continue to be fertile by producing eggs. If both ovaries are removed, this suddenly decreases the hormone levels and must be treated accordingly.

Should Your Ovaries Be Removed During a Hysterectomy?

If you are diagnosed with cancer, your ovaries might be removed because the hormones they secrete may encourage additional cancer growth. They also might be removed in severe cases of endometriosis. Again, the hormones they produce are responsible for endometriosis involving the ovary.

With the exception of cancer, the advantages and disadvantages of removing the ovaries (and the fallopian tubes) remain controversial. Some doctors believe that the ovaries should be removed when women are close to menopause and their ovarian function is diminishing anyway. Basically, it is a preventive measure that will reduce the risk of developing ovarian cancer later.

For women who are further away from menopause, there are more risks associated with removing healthy ovaries. Ovaries will continue to function after the uterus is removed. The ovaries produce hormones that protect against other serious diseases, such as cardiovascular disease and osteoporosis. Even as ovarian function begins to diminish, small amounts of hormones will still be released until they slowly taper off. Muscle and fat cells turn testosterone into circulating estrogen, in turn protecting against heart disease and osteoporosis.

Studies have shown that women whose ovaries are removed develop fewer breast cancers and their risk of ovarian cancer is almost entirely eliminated, but they are more likely to develop heart disease than women who keep their ovaries and more likely to die as a result of the heart disease. "If you take out the ovaries, the risk of ovarian cancer goes to zero," explains Dr. William Parker, a staff gynecologist at Santa

Monica–UCLA Medical Center in Los Angeles, "but you may lose the protection against heart disease and the prevention of osteoporosis." Also, some studies show intact ovaries may aid in preventing dementia as well.

Even though these studies were done on women going through traditional menopause, the results can inform your decision making. While your ovaries may not be functioning perfectly, they aren't, except in rare cases, diseased. Keeping healthy organs intact is ideal, if possible. Take your time, and explore all your options. Be well informed, and make your decision based on what is right for you with the help of your surgeon and health care team.

How Surgical Menopause Differs from Natural Menopause or Ovarian Insufficiency

> I had my hysterectomy two and a half years ago, when I was forty-three. The doctor told me I would go through menopause and have hot flashes, but she never told me about the awful mood swings I would experience. I immediately went on hormones, but those took a good four weeks or so to start working. I yelled at my husband all the time, or I bawled my eyes out. I was so moody. It would have been easier if I had known what to expect for those first few weeks.
>
> —Lauren

Surgical menopause happens with the removal of both ovaries in women who have not yet started to experience menopause or ovarian insufficiency. Because the ovaries are the main source of estrogen, progesterone, and androgens, hormone levels fall drastically when the ovaries are removed. Symptoms can occur immediately and include hot flashes, night sweats, vaginal dryness, palpitations, mood swings, depression, fatigue, and changes in sexual desire.

Major differences between surgical and natural menopause include:

- Surgical menopause occurs very suddenly—periods one day and menopause the next, unlike natural menopause, which occurs much more gradually over the course of many years.
- Surgical menopause typically results in much more intense symptoms.

- Surgical menopause involves recovering from major surgery, so time is needed to heal both physically and mentally and adjust to what just happened.

The Hysterectomy Surgical Procedure

Hysterectomy is the second most common operation performed on women in the United States. Approximately one out of every three American women will have a hysterectomy by age sixty. In recent years, the number of hysterectomies performed on women in their thirties and forties has been increasing. In fact, 55 percent of all hysterectomies are performed on women aged thirty-five to forty-nine. Even though there is a lot of talk about hysterectomies, the impact on younger women is usually ignored. As a result, it isn't a popular topic of discussion among younger women and thus women remain uninformed.

If you are one of the women who must have this type of surgery, what should you expect in terms of the surgery?

Questions to Ask Your Doctor About the Surgery
- What surgical approach will you use? (Laparoscopic, abdominal, vaginal, etc.)
- What side effects can I expect from the surgery?
- What kind of bleeding should I expect?
- What type of incision will I have, and what type of sutures will you use?
- How long will I be in the hospital?
- When can I resume my normal activities (work, child care, etc.)?
- What types of pain medication or other prescriptions will you prescribe after the surgery?
- What limitations will I have on sexual activity, and for how long?
- What will happen to my ovaries?
- Are there any other options that will let me leave my ovaries intact?
- What types of nonsurgical alternatives are currently available?
- What will happen if I don't have the surgery?
- What types of complications should I expect?
- How will this surgery affect my hormones?
- What if I want to have children?

BEFORE SURGERY

I had what I considered a very enlightened OB-GYN who discussed the operation and what I could expect following it quite thoroughly. He said that in his experience many women tended to experience exactly what they had been led to believe would happen. If the formative culture assumed that a woman without ovaries and womb was a sexless being, then the woman was more likely to feel negative than one who had never been told anything of the sort. As it turns out, I had not really ever discussed hysterectomy with anyone and my feelings had not been influenced one way or another. I am so grateful that I had time to process what the hysterectomy would mean to me before the surgery. I went into training for my operation, eating in a very healthy way and taking extra vitamin E for healing. I was up and about the following day and felt better than I had for years.

—Elsie

A hysterectomy is an inpatient procedure performed in a hospital setting. Before your surgery, your doctor will order a number of blood and urine tests. An enema is sometimes given to clean out your bowels before the surgery. Also, the abdominal and pelvic areas may be shaved and cleaned in order to prepare for surgery. You should also meet with an anesthesiologist to evaluate any special needs or conditions you have that might affect the anesthesia. Start eating soft foods three days before the surgery. On the night before the operation, you should eat a light meal and then have nothing to eat or drink for about twelve hours prior to your scheduled surgery.

KNOW YOUR HORMONE LEVELS

If you are scheduled for a hysterectomy, it is imperative to have a complete hormonal blood workup. That way there is a baseline to go by when determining your hormonal needs. You can look back at those tests, see what the levels were when you felt normal, and try to achieve those levels again with the right hormones. Because hormones fluctuate, talk to your health care provider about the timing of hormone testing.

Doctors, nurses, and women who have "been there" will all have experiences and advice for your recovery. How to remember everything?

Buy a notebook small enough to keep in your purse. As questions or tips strike you, write them down in there. As Maggie says, "I have carried it with me everywhere for the past three weeks, and it is worth its weight in gold!"

DURING SURGERY

Depending on the exact surgical method, the entire procedure should take somewhere between one and three hours. Regardless of the approach, the procedure involves separating the uterus from the ligaments and tissue that hold it in place. Once separated, it is then removed. Afterward, the instruments are removed and the incisions are closed. Laparoscopic incisions may be closed with absorbable sutures and sterile tape, while surgical incisions will be held together with staples and sutures that will be removed a couple of weeks later by your doctor.

TUMMY BANDS

This is an elastic, stretchy wrap that is wrapped around and around the abdomen, similar to an Ace bandage for a sprained ankle. Some doctors routinely wrap their hysterectomy patients with them after surgery, but ask beforehand if you should bring your own. Some brands even include a cooling gel pack to ease postoperative pain.

AFTER SURGERY

The best advice I never got: have a family member there as much as possible to see that you get what you are supposed to get at the scheduled time. I can't stress this enough. Having someone with you all the time means they will make sure you get your pain medications when you need them and not after the pain becomes miserable.

—Liz

After your surgery, you will feel some discomfort. If you had an abdominal hysterectomy, this discomfort will include the location of the incision. A typical hospital stay varies from same day to a few days depending on the type of surgery and any complications.

While you are in the hospital, ask for a recommendation for a stool softener. Having a bowel movement can be a little uncomfortable at first. Drink lots of water, and avoid foods like chocolate and dairy products, which may cause constipation.

AT HOME

Don't put yourself in a situation where you have to climb the stairs every day, at least for the first ten days. Consider buying (used is cheaper) or renting the following medical equipment to make the recovery much easier:

- A hospital table that easily wheels away from the bed but can also straddle the bed. This will allow you to read, use the computer, and eat without putting any pressure on your stomach or twisting around.
- Toilet hand-hold bars (there are temporary ones that rest on the toilet base; no need to attach them to the wall) to allow you to lower and raise yourself with your arms.
- A "grabber" that enables you to reach and pick up items on the floor or nearby.
- A walker with a seat for assistance getting into and out of bed and for the shower.
- Spa bags you can heat in the microwave or cool in the fridge, including a long, narrow one to cover the area of the incision (with a sheet between the spa bag and the incision).
- Wedge pillows, available at the local bed and bath store, which make sitting in bed much more comfortable.
- A body pillow or a large stuffed animal to hold on to.

Buy a short nightgown and robe of a silky material, both above knee length. That way you won't get all wrapped up in your nightclothes. Pajamas are not comfortable against the incision for the first two weeks.

What Can Younger Women Expect After Hysterectomy and/or Oophorectomy?

These surgeries do require a hospital stay and recovery at home. Women who have the necessary support at home as well as those who are generally physically fit can usually be released sooner. Overall recovery time varies, depending on the type of surgery and recovery speed, but it is safe to expect to take it easy for at least six weeks. Your doctor will tell you to avoid anything strenuous, such as carrying or lifting anything. This extensive recovery period can be difficult if you have a busy job or are caring for young children, so it is important to make appropriate arrangements beforehand.

Prepare for blood-stained discharge from your vagina for a few weeks. This usually stops after six weeks, at which time you will be able to resume your regular activities, including work and sexual intercourse. Ideally, you should not drive for about four weeks, until everything has had a chance to heal.

Though hysterectomies are relatively routine, the risk of complications does exist. One is reaction to the anesthesia. Blood clots can also form in the legs and can become very serious if they spread throughout the body. Also, because the reproductive organs are so close to the bowels and bladder, these systems can be damaged, requiring additional surgery later to correct them. In fact, almost half of women who undergo a hysterectomy develop a kidney or bladder infection following surgery. In some cases, especially with radical hysterectomies, the sensory nerves can be cut, resulting in the loss of the ability to feel the need to urinate and to control bladder function.

As with all surgeries, there is a risk of excess bleeding and/or infections. Some women will require a blood transfusion, especially if they suffer from preexisting anemia; infections are usually successfully treated with antibiotics. Many surgeons now routinely order antibiotics prior to surgery. In order to lessen the chance that an infection will occur, one should refrain from activities such as having intercourse, using tampons, douching, swimming, and taking baths for at least four weeks after the surgery.

What Happens Next?

Young women who have their reproductive organs surgically removed are thrust headlong into menopause. It is no surprise that this is very difficult for most of them. Instead of having years to gradually adjust to their symptoms and changing bodies, they have minimal time to prepare.

Young women who have had hysterectomies experience a wide range of symptoms related to ovarian sufficiency—from hot flashes to emotional issues to skin problems. The types of symptoms and their severity largely depend on which type of surgery was performed. While we talk about these symptoms and how best to cope throughout this book, a major concern among women with surgically induced menopause seems to revolve around sexuality and family building. As a result, we want to briefly touch on these topics now, with more to come in later chapters.

Young women are often afraid that this type of reproductive surgery will ruin their sex lives. Unfortunately, there is not much research about these topics, and most of the research that is available involves much older women. Still, there is no reason to believe you can't continue to have a healthy and fulfilling sex life. The biggest predictor of your sexuality after your operation was your preoperative sexual activity. Many women report no change in the way they feel sexually. In fact, many are able to enjoy sex more, since what was causing the pain or bleeding before is now gone. Think carefully about your sexuality and discuss your concerns with both your partner and health care provider.

Another major concern is family building. Many young women who have their reproductive organs removed may not have started their family building yet. Even for those who do already have children, it might be difficult for them to accept the realization that they will never carry another child or have another genetically related child. Today, there are many family-building options that young women can pursue.

First, young women can consider having their eggs frozen if they are going to have their ovaries removed. Egg freezing, while still considered experimental by some, has made great strides recently. Many fertility clinics are having success in freezing the eggs of women who want to retain their ability to have a genetically related child. If this interests you, make sure you go to a reputable clinic that has proven success with egg freezing. If you already have a partner (or if you want to consider a sperm donor), you can have your eggs retrieved and then fertilized with sperm to create embryos. These embryos can be frozen. Frozen embryos tend to fare better than frozen eggs. These embryos can be transferred to your uterus through IVF whenever you are ready. If you don't have an intact uterus, you can utilize a gestational surrogate.

For women who have already had their reproductive organs removed without considering these options, you can look into egg donation and surrogacy. More than ten thousand families turn to egg donation and several hundred others use surrogates each year to build their families. Most fertility clinics offer egg donor programs or you can opt to find your egg donor through an independent agency. There are also many agencies and reproductive attorneys that can assist you in locating a surrogate. Adoption is a great choice for many families. In any case, be prepared to discuss your family building options with your health care provider as you plan your surgery. While these are all great ways for bringing a child into your life, research and advance planning can help ensure a successful experience.

Sometimes it is impossible to avoid a hysterectomy or other surgeries that affect your reproductive organs, but with proper education and preparation, young women can learn to maximize their chances of living a full and healthy life. The more information you have at the beginning, the better you will be able to prepare for the future.

7

Cancer and Ovarian Function

When I was first diagnosed with Hodgkin's disease, I was told by my oncologist that the treatment would in no way affect my ovaries, etc. I was given a letter-type thing which outlined what Hodgkin's was, what kind of treatment I would be having, and how this would affect me, so that I could show my friends at school to explain everything— and it says on it that "Kate will still be able to have babies after her treatment." This, together with the oncologist's assurances, meant that neither I or my parents gave my fertility a second thought. My periods continued right the way through my treatment (ten months), and then all of a sudden about six months or so after having finished my treatment I started getting hot flushes, and then my periods stopped. At my regular checkup with the oncologist I mentioned this and was referred to a gynecologist, who carried out an ultrasound and blood tests, then informed me, in a rather matter-of-fact way, that I would never be able to have children and that I should take the pill to stop me getting osteoporosis; she mentioned egg donation in passing, but nothing more.

—Kate

ABOUT ONE IN 333 GIRLS will develop cancer before her twentieth birthday. Currently, there are more than 500,000 young women who are survivors of cancer during childhood or their very early reproductive years. Additionally, more than 60,000 women of childbearing age are diagnosed with some type of cancer each year. Overall, cancer during childhood and young adulthood occurs about twice as often in women as in men. The most common types of childhood cancer include leukemia, brain cancer, soft-tissue cancer, non-Hodgkin's lymphoma, kidney and renal cancer, bone and joint cancer, and Hodgkin's lymphoma. The most common cancers among women of childbearing years seem to be breast cancer, colorectal cancer, lung cancer, uterine cancer, ovarian cancer, non-Hodgkin's lymphoma, pancreatic cancer, bladder cancer, leukemia, and stomach cancer. Although a diagnosis of cancer in childhood or young adulthood (ages twenty to forty-four) is still a relatively rare event, there are important consequences, including cancer's impact on ovarian function.

How Cancer and Cancer Treatment Affect Your Ovaries

Not all cancers and cancer treatments negatively impact the ovaries, but many do. Some cancers, such as thyroid cancer, have a relatively small chance of affecting your ovaries. With other cancers, such as breast cancer, the type of treatment varies and can affect your ovaries differently depending on the specific treatment protocol. Overall, cancers that are considered "high risk" result in more than 80 percent of patients experiencing a loss of ovarian function. For "intermediate risk," 20 to 80 percent of patients will have ovarian insufficiency. For "low risk," the statistic is less than 20 percent. For more information about your specific risk potential with regard to both the type of cancer you have and your specific treatment protocol, check out the Risk Calculator at www.fertilehope.org.

Fertile Hope is a nonprofit organization that offers fertility resources for cancer patients. You may visit www.fertilehope.org or contact them at 888-994-HOPE (4673). Along with information about treatment options and how to find a good health care provider, this organization provides excellent support and suggestions to help overcome some of the financial barriers you might meet.

Understand your individual risks concerning how your cancer and cancer treatment will affect you and your ovarian function. Certain cancer treatments, including chemotherapy and radiation, can be toxic to the ovaries, leading to both loss of hormone production and infertility. Unfortunately, having a period does not equate to ovarian function. Even patients who continue to have menstrual cycles usually have evidence of decreased ovarian function.

YOUR HEALTH CARE PROVIDER

A cancer diagnosis is frightening, and your first visit will probably be to whomever your primary care physician recommends. A second opinion is often very valuable, but you will want to see someone who specializes in the kind of cancer you have. An oncologist specializes in the diagnosis and treatment of malignancies. A medical oncologist has been board-certified in internal medicine, with a subspecialty in medical oncology. An oncologist usually specializes in a specific body system; for instance, a reproductive oncologist specializes in seeing patients with malignancies of the uterus, cervix, ovaries, and vagina. Also, you want to find a health care provider who is knowledgeable about cancer and your reproductive risk. Their area of expertise (called oncofertility) is fairly new yet growing.

Age and Ovarian Function

Age plays an important role in ovarian function for all women, regardless of cancer. As a woman ages, her ovaries produce fewer good-quality eggs until they stop making eggs altogether. This is when you go through menopause. Not surprisingly, at what age you undergo your cancer treatment has a lot to do with how your ovaries will respond. Higher doses and older ages at the time of treatment are both associated with greater damage. The younger you are at the time of cancer treatments, the more likely it is that your ovaries will continue to produce eggs after your treatment. In fact, girls and women past the age of puberty may be at greater risk than younger children, as the ovaries of younger girls can often tolerate higher doses of chemotherapy than the ovaries of women. Once you reach age thirty-five, you become much more vulnerable to ovarian insufficiency after chemotherapy. At age forty, this vulnerability increases even more.

Centers of Excellence in Cancer and Fertility

Fertile Hope (www.fertilehope.com) has identified the following hospitals and clinics as Centers of Excellence. These cancer facilities have demonstrated that they inform all patients about their reproductive risks; provide educational materials for health care providers, patients, and survivors; make referrals to appropriate fertility specialists; and when possible conduct research on cancer-related infertility, pregnancy after cancer, and/or parenthood after cancer.

- Abramson Cancer Center of the University of Pennsylvania (Pennsylvania)
- NYU Cancer Institute of the New York University Medical Center (New York)
- Robert H. Lurie Comprehensive Cancer Center of Northwestern University (Illinois)
- Stanford Comprehensive Cancer Center (California)
- Cleveland Clinic Taussig Cancer Institute (Ohio)
- Kimmel Cancer Center at Thomas Jefferson University (Pennsylvania)

Childhood Cancer

People don't want to hear that children grow up and have all these problems because they had cancer. I think that children who grow up now are going to be a lot healthier than I am, because they've improved the treatment. But the adult survivor of childhood cancer is a face of cancer that needs to be better represented and acknowledged.

—Rebecca, a twenty-seven-year Hodgkin's survivor

Types of Cancer Treatments

I spent most of the time since being diagnosed and now denying the situation—I took the pills and fielded questions from the doctors, and I managed to convince myself that if they'd been wrong in the first instance about my chemo not affecting me, then why couldn't they be wrong about my ovaries, too?

—Anna

It seems particularly unfair that not only do you have to deal with cancer, but chemotherapy, radiation, and surgery can all affect ovarian function and fertility. The risks of chemotherapy depend on the type and dose of the drug and how it is given. The risks of radiation therapy again depend on the dose of radiation and the area of the body that is irradiated. Surgery on the reproductive organs or around those organs can damage the ovaries as well.

CHEMOTHERAPY

Chemotherapy is the general term used for any treatment involving the use of chemical agents to kill existing cancer cells and stop the cancer cells from growing. More than half of all people diagnosed with cancer receive some sort of chemotherapy. Chemotherapy medications are extremely potent, and virtually all chemotherapy drugs affect a woman's ability to become pregnant. Because the research in this area is very limited, it is difficult to know how any individual woman will be affected. Still, there are a number of key points that we do know.

Ovarian insufficiency due to chemotherapy medications may be temporary. In other words, ovulation and your menstrual cycle may stop during treatment and while you are recovering from treatment and may start again once treatment is over. It can take anywhere from a few months or up to a year or longer for your periods to return. The effects of chemotherapy on ovarian function seem to be related to the dosage. Women who receive higher doses of chemotherapy medications experience a greater impact on their ovaries than do those on lower-dose regimens.

Some chemotherapy medications, especially those that belong to a group called alkylating agents, cause more damage to the ovaries than others. It is important to remember that chemotherapy medications are rarely given alone. Instead, they are used together in different combinations and in different dosages. And those combinations and dosages can have different effects on the ovaries.

On average, about half of women under the age of thirty-five get their periods back after they finish their chemotherapy treatment. Some of them may be able to become pregnant without difficulty. However, others will have difficulty, especially if the treatment damaged the immature eggs in the ovaries. The number of immature eggs left in the ovaries influences the rate of ovarian function decline. The fewer immature eggs you have, the less your ovaries are able to function properly.

Your ovaries control ovulation and dictate your menstrual cycle. This means that if you have a regular period, some of your eggs are maturing and being released. However, this number may be much smaller than if you had not had chemotherapy. As a result, your egg supply may be depleted at a much faster rate than other women's.

Even if you are ovulating, the chemotherapy might have caused some genetic damage to your developing eggs. This damage may contribute to an increased risk of birth defects. It is important to use birth control assiduously during your entire treatment in order to minimize this risk. Once your treatment is completed, most doctors suggest waiting at least six months to recover from the lingering side effects of treatment. This time will allow some of your eggs to repair themselves from being exposed to the highly potent chemotherapy medications.

BREAST CANCER MEDICATIONS

Taxanes are a group of chemotherapy medications that are very effective in treating breast cancer. These medications include Taxol (paclitaxel) and Taxotere (docetaxel).

Chemotherapy medications that have a high risk of affecting the ovaries:
Cytoxan (cyclophosphamide)
Matulane (procarbazine)

Chemotherapy medications that have a medium risk of affecting the ovaries:
Platinol (cisplatin)
Adriamycin (doxorubicin)

Chemotherapy medications that have a low risk of affecting the ovaries:
Amethopterin (methotrexate)
Adrucil (5-fluorouracil or 5-FU)
Oncovin (vincristine)

RADIATION THERAPY

Radiation therapy is used to treat cancer by itself or in combination with other forms of treatment such as surgery or chemotherapy. At very high doses (many times greater than those used for X-ray exams), radiation can kill cancer cells and shrink tumors. More than half of all cancer patients receive some type of radiation therapy as part of their overall treatment. Radiation therapy can be given externally or internally. In external radiation therapy, an external beam is administered just like a normal X-ray. The radiation machines deliver intense treatments with pinpoint accuracy. Internal radiation therapy involves placing radioactive substances, such as cesium, iridium, and iodine, near the cancerous cells or into the affected area of the body.

There is still little research available assessing the impact of radiation therapy on the ovaries. The location of the radiation therapy is the most important factor in how it will affect the ovaries. The closer the radiation occurs to the ovaries, the greater its impact. Women who have received abdominal or pelvic radiation have an increased risk of damage to their reproductive organs, including both the uterus and ovaries. Even low doses of radiation to this area can affect ovarian function. For women receiving radiation treatment, especially to the pelvic region, it is important to shield the ovaries as much as possible to minimize the effects. In many cases, if one ovary does not receive radiation, the ovarian function may be maintained. If both ovaries are exposed to radiation, the chances are decreased.

CANCER SURGERY

Surgery is often used to treat a variety of different cancers, especially female cancers. The effects of this surgery on ovarian function can depend on the specific type of surgery performed. For instance, removal of both ovaries and/or the uterus will permanently affect a woman's ability to get pregnant. Though an operation on the cervix, vagina, or vulva will impact a woman's chances of having a child, more conservative fertility-preserving techniques can be considered if appropriate. For example, an abdominal radical trachelectomy (ART) is used to treat cervical cancer. It generally does not directly impact ovarian function and leaves the uterus intact. Women are still able to utilize their own eggs, carry a child, and give birth via cesarean section.

BONE MARROW AND STEM CELL TRANSPLANTS

Bone marrow and stem cell transplants use high-dose chemotherapy and radiation to destroy cancer cells. These types of procedures are typically used to treat patients diagnosed with leukemia, lymphoma, and multiple myeloma and sometimes solid breast and ovarian cancer tumors. Side effects of these lifesaving therapies include the destruction of normal cells in the body, including reproductive cells. Bone marrow and stem cell transplants infuse healthy cells back into your body. For women, ovarian insufficiency is almost a certain side effect of bone marrow and stem cell transplants. This can be temporary or permanent. Because little research exists about fertility after bone marrow and stem cell transplants, it is impossible to predict beforehand how the transplant will affect your ovaries or your fertility.

PRESERVING OVARIAN FUNCTION

While cancer treatments always run the risk of diminishing ovarian function, a number of options can be considered to lessen the impact on your fertility. However, none of these issues will completely prevent the progress of ovarian insufficiency. Once your cancer has been successfully diagnosed, you will need to talk with your health care provider about maintaining good hormonal health no matter your fertility.

PROTECTING THE OVARIES

If you are receiving radiation treatments, there are a few procedures that will help decrease the radiation to your ovaries. Your health care provider can place external shields over the site of your ovaries during the radiation treatment. Alternatively, your doctor can decide to surgically move ovaries out of the radiation field. Once treatment is completed, the ovaries are moved back to their original position. This process is called *ovarian transposition*.

EMBRYO CRYOPRESERVATION

Before you undergo cancer treatments, you can have your eggs removed and fertilized with sperm from your husband or partner or a sperm donor. Embryos can be cryopreserved (frozen) for many years. You can then decide to have them transferred back to your uterus or use a gestational surrogate. While embryo cryopreservation is probably the easiest and most straightforward option for extending your fertility, you will need to carefully consider this option for several reasons. First, you want to make sure that any delay in treatment needed to remove your eggs won't interfere with conquering your cancer. Similarly, because hormones will be needed to stimulate your ovaries to produce more eggs, you want to ensure that those hormones won't aggravate the cancer. Also, decide how you feel about having frozen embryos, especially regarding the long term. Finally, fertility treatments are expensive. Expect to pay about $15,000 for removing your eggs, $5,000 for each attempt at pregnancy, $30,000 or more for a gestational surrogate, and about $1,000 each year to store your embryos.

EGG FREEZING

While freezing unfertilized eggs is still considered investigational, many advances have been made in this area. Before you decide to freeze your eggs, talk to your doctor about the realistic chances of success. And go to a reputable clinic with significant experience with egg freezing. Even under the best of circumstances, egg freezing is not as successful as freezing embryos. There are still many unanswered questions about egg freezing: How long can eggs be frozen? How many eggs should be frozen? Additionally, how will egg freezing affect your cancer treatments in terms of delaying treatment or the hormones used?

Egg freezing may be an option for women who do not yet have a partner and want to preserve their eggs for later use. Again, egg freezing is expensive—about $15,000 to $20,000 to obtain and freeze the eggs plus another $15,000 to $20,000 for each IVF attempt. And don't forget the storage fees to the tune of about $1,000 per year.

OVARIAN TISSUE FREEZING

The first birth in the United States after ovarian tissue was removed, frozen, and later implanted occurred in September 2005, to Ann Dauer, then thirty-three. Being able to freeze her ovary gave Ann hope during her stem cell transplant to fight non-Hodgkin's lymphoma in 2002.

After her ovary was removed and frozen, she said, she would lie in the hospital bed thinking, "I've done every step I can to keep all my dreams alive."

The ovary can be removed, tissue carefully dissected with microsurgery, frozen, and subsequently transplanted back to the woman after she has been cured of the cancer. As described by Dr. Sherman Silber of the Infertility Center of St. Louis, "all of a woman's eggs can be found in the thin one-millimeter outer layer of the ovary, while the inside of the ovary is simply a pulp of blood vessels with no specific organization or function other than to feed the eggs and follicles that are located on the periphery. This structure makes it possible for an entire ovary to be removed and the periphery dissected off microsurgically. The ovarian tissue is then put through a computer-controlled, gradual freezing process. This procedure is very new, and little is known about its overall outcomes. Ovarian tissue is removed during an outpatient surgical procedure and frozen for future transplantation back into your body. The goal is to preserve immature eggs and tissue that produces female hormones to potentially preserve fertility."

OVARIAN SUPPRESSION

Some researchers are suggesting that you can suppress ovarian function during cancer treatments to help protect your eggs from damage. Right now, this research is highly controversial. While it seems like a good idea to temporarily stop ovarian function during treatment, some doctors are concerned that the drugs used for ovarian suppression may interfere with the treatment's ability to kill the cancer cells. Cancer treatments, especially chemotherapy medications, are most effective against cancer cells when they are actively growing. Ovarian suppression uses hormones called gonadotropin-releasing hormone (GnRH) antagonists to suppress the ovaries. The most common GnRH antagonists are Zoladex (goserelin) and Lupron (leuprolide). When GnRH is blocked, no ovulation takes place. Unfortunately, these hormones can also stop or slow the growth of cancer cells as well, which may make the cells less sensitive to the chemotherapy medications.

MEDICATIONS

Some research has shown that women who take oral contraceptives (birth control pills) during chemotherapy may retain ovarian function following treatment. However, since this method involves hormones, it is not recommended for women with cancers that are sensitive to hormones (especially breast cancer).

Hormone Therapy (HT) After Cancer Treatments

I'm thirty-nine and was diagnosed with rectal cancer last year and had to undergo radiochemotherapy, which of course destroyed my ovaries and put me into premature menopause. It's been a few months already, and I have to complete a four-and-a-half-month course of chemo. It was a horrible thing to learn I was going into menopause suddenly, but it's also so hard to know I can't begin treatment for that until after the chemo is done.

—Leah

Young women who experience acute loss of ovarian function due to their cancer treatments will struggle with estrogen deficiency. Taking HT after cancer treatment is a very difficult decision for many young women. Since nothing is absolute, you will have to consider both the benefits and the risks. For younger women, the benefits can be health-protective, possibly preventing other serious health concerns later in life, such as osteoporosis and heart disease, as well as minimizing the symptoms associated with diminishing ovarian function. Risks include the sensitivity of certain types of cancers to hormones, perhaps increasing your chances that the cancer will return.

Unfortunately, there is little information available regarding the impact of HT on young cancer patients. The final decision will depend on what type of cancer it was, how advanced it was, and how aggressive it was. If your cancer was at a low state, not very aggressive, and not sensitive to estrogen, and other methods of treating low hormone levels have failed, taking HT might be an option for you. Remember, whatever your decision is, it should be reassessed periodically; research in this field is rapidly changing.

Talking with Your Health Care Provider

Doctors are making tremendous strides in cancer research each day. More and more people are not only surviving cancer but thriving afterward. Still, recovery from cancer can take many years, so many patients do not feel physically or psychologically ready to consider family building right away. But ovarian function affects much more than just your reproductive capacity. As discussed in earlier chapters, the ovaries control hormones that are vital for many different aspects of healthy living. Despite your family-building goals, a thorough pretreatment discussion of expectations and options is essential to preserving your fertility and helping you plan effectively for the future.

Questions to Ask Your Doctor About Cancer and Fertility

- What are the short-term and long-term effects on the ovaries from cancer treatment?
- What is the risk of permanent ovarian failure with the treatments recommended for my type, stage, and grade of cancer?
- Are there any other treatment options that can be considered that do not pose as high a risk but are equally effective?
- What are the options for preserving my ovarian function?
- Will any of these options make my cancer treatments less effective or increase the risk that my cancer will return?
- Can I become pregnant while receiving cancer treatments?
- How long must I wait after treatment before I can try to become pregnant?
- Is it appropriate for me to consult a fertility specialist or a reproductive endocrinologist?
- Where can I get more information and support about cancer and ovarian function?
- What are the long-term implications of having diminished ovarian function?
- What are the plans for my long-term care?

PART THREE

Treatment Options

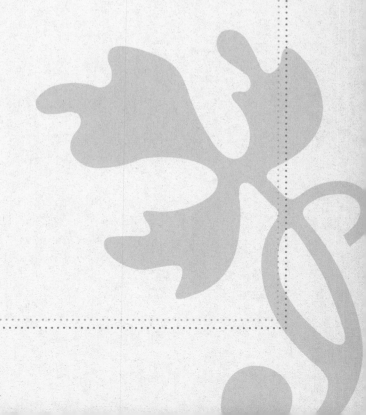

8

Your Health Care Providers

I am more than my ovaries, dammit. Every time I visit my doctor, he doesn't bother to look at me. He comes in the exam room, reviews my latest blood hormone levels, and tells me what medication changes he wants to make. The last time I asked a question about a new symptom, he said something about how "Now you know what women have been going through for thousands of years." What a slap in the face!

—Teresa

Integrated Care

The concept of integrated care is fairly new in modern medicine. The theory is that an integrated care practitioner is committed to treating all of you—not just your disease. Since ovarian deficiency affects so many aspects of your health, an integrative approach is important. Sometimes this approach includes complementary and alternative treatment as well as lifestyle changes. It is healing-oriented medicine that takes account of the whole person (body, mind, and spirit), including all aspects of care:

- Evidence-based care means patients make informed decisions based on the best available data on the efficacy and safety of all treatment options.
- Whole-person care should not only attend to the patient's physical aspects but also address the patient's emotional,

psychological, spiritual, social, and cultural needs and dimensions.

- Relationship and patient-centered care is designed to recognize that the relationship between the health care provider and the patient is of fundamental importance. The health care provider therefore strives to respect the wishes and experience of the individual and encourages the patient to become an active partner in his or her own care.
- Self-care is based on the belief that health care providers should be teachers who facilitate a desire and ability for patients to care for themselves to both prevent and alleviate illness. Additionally, providers can best serve the needs of others by embodying a philosophy of self-care and being truly attentive to their own health and well-being.

Another reason integrated care is a wise approach is a growing emphasis on patient satisfaction as a legitimate outcome of care, and an awareness is needed on the part of insurers and practitioners that integrated care can offer a broad array of options that may significantly enhance healing and promote more active patient participation in health maintenance and compliance.

Getting a Diagnosis

I'll never forget that afternoon when the nurse called me. I had gone to my OB/GYN, who ordered tests, never mentioning any possibilities for why my periods suddenly stopped. I was home alone on the day before my twenty-seventh birthday, and the nurse called, telling me I was in premature menopause. She told me I was lucky not to have to worry about periods anymore. I spent the afternoon looking online for information, and I was terrified and overwhelmed. Heart disease, osteoporosis, no kids, and what the hell was an atrophied vagina? I went to bed and cried for hours. I hated that doctor for handling my diagnosis so badly.

—Lana

A diagnosis of ovarian insufficiency needs to come from a physician in person. The nature of the condition requires lab tests to confirm a suspected cause. Physicians often forget, however, that how patients handle a diagnosis can be significantly impacted by how their health care providers give it. As Lana's story shows, the doctor's attitude in communicating the diagnosis is important.

Another young woman describes her diagnosis at fifteen: "I remember the physician saying, 'Maybe you could marry a divorcé who already has children, for you have no future at all.' That I have come a long way from all that is a different story, but today after eleven years, when I look back, I see a scared teenager sitting inside a cramped room with her parents. I was grappling with the enormity of what has just been said, being very brave, trying not to cry. I do not think I understood fully what he told me." She continues, "there is a certain insensitivity seen in most physicians, which can at times be argued in favor of by them saying that otherwise they would never be able to carry on their work, but look at it from the individual's point of view, in her prime, whose potential has been snatched away from her before she has even realized it . . . she needs hand-holding."

Cara tells a different story: "About three months ago, I sat in my new doctor's office explaining to her how I kept going hot and cold, that I hadn't been feeling right for a long time, that my migraines had been getting worse, how my emotions went from one extreme to another, how I was not sleeping very well, and how I kept having really bad depressive bouts over nothing. I felt I was going to get some answers, as she seemed very thorough. She was the first doctor to actually send me for any kind of tests.

"I found myself once again sitting in her office, nervous as hell. When she spoke calmly, with such a soft and reassuring voice, I started to feel a little bit more trusting, simply because I actually felt like she cared. We spoke about the results and why she had asked for them to be done. Then she explained that there was a problem with my hormones. I thought maybe my balance had changed and she was going to suggest a different pill, but obviously not. I was postmenopausal. *At the age of twenty!*

"When she asked me if I understood what this meant, I knew one thing: that I couldn't have kids. I'm twenty. How can I not have kids? I sat there and cried. I thought she was going to cry with me, she was so apologetic and said she wished she did not have to give me such news. But she helped me find a good specialist and is encouraging me to not to give up."

An effective health care provider will:

- Make the diagnosis promptly and accurately.
- Inform the patient of the diagnosis in a sensitive and supportive manner.
- Counsel the patient in a way that validates her emotional concerns and helps her to maintain control of her physical and emotional health.
- Explain hormone therapy and other appropriate treatments.
- Assess and continue to reassess for the presence of other disorders related to spontaneous primary ovarian insufficiency.

The doctor should be the one communicating with the patient and not relegate that responsibility to staff. The physician must strive to be sympathetic and communicate face-to-face, not by phone. He or she must also be willing to thoroughly explain the diagnosis, acknowledge the areas that he or she knows little about, and allow the patient time to process the information, knowing that follow-up appointments will probably be necessary for her to adapt to her new reality.

Finding a Good Health Care Provider

There are many providers who are experienced with menopause but very few who have specific skills in working with women who are going through ovarian insufficiency. If you are not considering pregnancy, you can start with talking to your regular gynecologist. Patients need to realize that most providers do not see a large number of patients with this type of diagnosis in their practice and therefore may not have sufficient clinical experience to be able to answer questions and/or provide an up-to-date evaluation of their condition. Dr. Michael Heard of the Women's Specialists of Houston explains: "Searching for the most informed providers through resources like POI/POF support groups may help inform and educate patients and point them in the right direction, so they can get the care and attention they deserve. They must be properly evaluated and counseled about the disorder and followed closely by their provider. It is important to see someone who is trained to take care of patients with this condition and counsel them about future risks, including the possibility of autoimmune disease, need for HT, and future fertility concerns. Many patients are being diagnosed by FSH alone and offered HT and egg donation without other diagnostic testing or follow-up."

Since coping with diminishing ovarian function may last several years, you want to find a health care provider you feel comfortable talking to throughout this process. Be open and honest about any new symptoms or concerns. Diminishing ovarian function can affect many different areas of your life, including physical, emotional, and sexual. Because you may not have any friends who are going through this experience, it is critical that you seek support and develop a good relationship with your health care provider, as well as seek additional support.

Dr. Lawrence explains, "Patients with spontaneous premature ovarian failure benefit greatly from a solid and ongoing relationship with a sensitive and well-informed health care practitioner. The time constraints currently imposed on clinicians can make caring for a woman with premature ovarian failure a frustrating experience, for both patient and clinician."

MAKING THE MOST OF YOUR DOCTOR VISIT

- Document and prioritize your symptoms, including how often you have them and how severe they are.
- Learn about hormone therapy in general ahead of time.
- Document your family health history and ask about how your diagnosis will impact the rest of your family and their risk of experiencing ovarian insufficiency and related concerns.
- Bring someone with you to provide support and another set of ears.
- Come to your doctor's office with a list of questions prepared.

Types of Health Care Providers

In the course of your lifetime dealing with ovarian insufficiency issues, you will deal with a variety of types of health care providers. Just whom you'll see depends on your health insurance, your geographical location (or where you are willing to travel) and your particular concerns.

WHICH TYPE OF DOCTOR SHOULD I SEE?

Because ovarian insufficiency affects your health in many ways, you might need to see various health care providers about your concerns. Some examples include:

Type of Provider	What They Do
Cardiologist	Helps you prevent and manage heart disease
Dermatologist	Deals with skin-related issues, as well as hair and nail problems
Endocrinologist	Interested in your hormones and endocrine system
General practitioner/Internist	Assists you with your overall general health concerns and physical well-being
Geneticist	Identifies genetic abnormalities or concerns
Gynecologist	Concentrates on your reproductive health and reproductive organs
Orthopedist	Specializes in bone concerns, especially as the result of osteoporosis
Psychiatrist	Works with you regarding your mental health concerns
Reproductive endocrinologist	Focuses on fertility and helping you have a baby

NORTH AMERICAN MENOPAUSE SOCIETY CERTIFIED
MENOPAUSE PRACTITIONER PROGRAM

If you are looking for a health care provider who can provide optimal meno-pause-related health care, consider looking at those who are certified by the North American Menopause Society Certified Menopause Practitioner Pro-gram. Candidates must be licensed health care practitioners, including physicians, physician assistants, nurse practitioners, nurses, pharmacists, and psychologists. They are also required to pass an examination consisting of 100 multiple-choice questions in English, developed through a combined effort of qualified subject matter experts and testing professionals who have constructed it in accordance with the examination content outline. The NAMS Menopause Practitioner cre-dential is valid for three years. The credential can be maintained by either passing a new examination or submitting appropriate continuing medical education credits that demonstrate ongoing education. For a listing of current NAMS Menopause Practitioners, go to www.menopause.org.

Questions to Ask Your Doctor About Ovarian Insufficiency

- How much experience do you have treating women in my situation?
- Can my symptoms be caused by any condition other than primary ovarian insufficiency or early menopause?
- How will you properly diagnose my primary ovarian insufficiency?
- What is causing my primary ovarian insufficiency?
- What type of hormone replacement therapy do you recommend and why? What are the advantages and side effects associated with this therapy?
- What else can I do to control my symptoms?
- Am I at risk of any long-term health concerns, such as osteoporosis, heart disease, or cancer?
- Where can I go for emotional support?
- How can I tell my friends and family about my diagnosis?
- What are your plans for my long-term care?

FOLLOW-UP CARE

Make sure to schedule a follow-up appointment once you receive a diagnosis. Doing so will allow you to process some of the information you have received and give you an opportunity to do your own research and come up with a list of questions you would like to address.

A New Kind of Clinic

Because ovarian insufficiency affects many aspects of a woman's life and encompasses much more than fertility, Stanford University has developed the first multidisciplinary program for women with ovarian insufficiency. This program is led by a wonderful team of doctors (mostly women, we might add) who have a great deal of experience specifically treating women for concerns related to ovarian insufficiency. Integrative care and general health concerns are priorities.

This clinic is also actively working to improve the quality of health for women with ovarian insufficiency through participating in a wide range of research efforts. This clinic also offers a full range of services. As Medical Director Dr. Valerie Baker explains, "I believe that it is critically important to carefully review each person's individual situation, so that we can provide the care that will give the best chance of having a healthy baby. Although I provide clear recommendations about evaluation and treatment, I feel that it is also very important to provide information about choices, so that people can have input into making the decisions that are right for them." For more information about this

innovative program, visit the program's Web site at www.stanfordivf
.com/poi.html.

Also, the federal government, through the National Institutes of
Health (NIH) has invested significant resources in studying women
with diminishing ovarian function. NIH doctors are conducting a clinical research program whose goal is to develop improved treatments for
women with ovarian insufficiency. These studies will also help doctors
and patients learn more about POI. Most important, this research is
clarifying how POI affects young women and how POI differs from
menopause.

> *Almost everything I found online redirected me to the National Institutes of
> Health (NIH) Web site, which I learned was the knowledge leader on the subject
> of premature ovarian failure. During the days that I stayed at NIH, I under-
> went extensive testing and monitoring. There, I found experts who care about
> women like me and are willing to make a difference. During the weeks leading
> up to and following my NIH trip, I was struggling to find inner peace within
> myself. It was difficult to sort through the many complicated emotions I was
> experiencing. I tried to develop an acceptance of the disease, but it was so hard.
> Still, being at the NIH was a godsend.*
>
> —Rebekah

The NIH Clinical Center is located in Bethesda, Maryland (about
nine miles north of Washington, D.C.), and is the world's largest hospital devoted to the research of both common and rare diseases. There is
no cost to participate in the POI program at NIH, and all participants
receive personalized care, free study-related medications, and a comprehensive clinical and laboratory evaluation. To find out more about this
program or to see if you qualify to participate, visit its Web site at http://
poi.nichd.nih.gov.

Get to Know Your Pharmacist

The pharmacist is probably the most underutilized health professional.
Where else can you stop by without an appointment and ask questions
about your medications? If you have any concerns or questions about
your medications (both prescription and over the counter), make sure
you talk to your pharmacist. Always let him or her know if you change

medications, are taking any new medications, or experience any side effects. If he or she can't help you, he or she probably knows where to turn. In some cases, a pharmacist is willing to make a call to your doctor's office on your behalf, which is usually quicker and much more effective than your trying to reach them on your own.

A World of Information

Another form of support is gaining information. While women can and do go online to find resources for education and support, it can be overwhelming to go through hundreds of Web pages, many of which are advertisements for supplements or other products. "When I was diagnosed," says Susan, "my doctor gave me pathetic menopause literature with drawings of elderly, gray-haired women on the front. I was thirty-two. The first line of the literature read, 'You can still live out your remaining years productively.' I almost burst into tears right then and there. He just said, 'Sorry, there is just no literature to give you for your condition.'" Educational handouts and a resource list of books and online resources, as well as information on support groups, can be valuable tools for a newly diagnosed patient.

Searching for "early menopause" on Google yields thousands of Web sites. And that doesn't include related terms such as hormone replacement therapy, bioidentical hormones, or hysterectomies. When you are facing a health issue such as ovarian insufficiency, the Internet can be a valuable place to begin. With all the online forums, blogs, and shopping sites, there are thousands of places to look for information.

How Reliable Is This Site?
Check to see if it has the HON logo. Health on the Net Foundation is the leading organization that promotes and guides the presentation of useful and reliable online medical and health information. HON is a nonprofit, nongovernmental organization that's even accredited by the United Nations. For more information, and a list of accredited sites, go to www.hon.ch.

Surfing the Internet can be helpful, but it can be misleading as well. After all, anyone can post anything online, regardless of whether it's true or based on best practices, or even if its safety is in doubt. Many of the sites are meant to look informative but are simply cleverly designed sales sites. But remember, just as ovarian insufficiency is not the same diagnosis as menopause, neither can the hundreds of sites claiming "menopause relief" in a bottle speak to your unique situation.

9

Medical Treatments

I'm on the estrogen patch, but I don't think the doctor gave me all the instructions. I wore it over my left eye for a week and made six people walk the plank . . . helped with the mood swings, but didn't do much for the hot flashes.

—Leigh Anne Jasheway-Bryant, author of
Not Guilty by Reason of Menopause

WE HEAR AN AWFUL lot about hormone therapy. Not too long ago, it was referred to as hormone replacement therapy, or HRT, and focused primarily on treating women who had natural menopause at a normal age. Today we tend to call it just hormone therapy, or HT for short, because we now understand that hormone therapy is applicable to a wider range of women, including those who experience surgical menopause or ovarian insufficiency.

Although there has been a lot of bad press lately about the dangers of hormone therapy, this doesn't necessarily apply to you. Women who experience natural, normally timed menopause may not need hormone therapy, but most experts agree that ovarian insufficiency experienced by younger women does require some type of hormone therapy. For these women, it is important to maintain the natural life cycle and menstrual cycle patterns of your hormones as much as possible. Hormone therapy is most effective when it is taken and stopped in ways that mimic natural and normal patterns. This chapter is meant to help you feel confident about your decisions so you can live a long and healthy life.

Hormone Therapy (HT)

One doctor said to me that there are two areas in the human body we don't yet fully understand. One of these is the brain. The other, of course, is women's hormonal system.

—Elisa

Since the human body makes many different types of hormones, it makes sense to believe that when a certain hormone is lacking, it should be replaced. We do this all the time. When you have an underactive thyroid gland, it is treated with the addition of thyroid hormones; diabetes is treated with insulin, and so on. The ovary is responsible for making estrogen, progesterone, and some testosterone (the male hormone), so these hormones must be supplemented when they begin to run low. "Doc, I'm down a quart of estrogen and a liter of progesterone. Fill 'er up."

Hormone therapy (HT) is prescribing hormones for women whose own hormone levels are low. It seems as though everyone has a different opinion about HT, including both medical professionals and the lay public. As new research emerges, the understanding of HT is also changing. Most of the debates in this area have centered on the specific use of estrogen and how a woman's body utilizes estrogen throughout her life.

Although most health care providers agree that women with ovarian insufficiency do benefit from HT, every woman is different with regard to her specific needs. As a result, it is important that each woman find the best method and dosage for her. Each component of HT (estrogen, progesterone, and testosterone) can be prescribed individually to effectively tailor the right mix of medications, especially in terms of dosages and regimens.

Unfortunately, this sometimes (okay, a lot of the time) requires some trial and error. Even once a good protocol has been established, it might need to be changed again and then again, as you get older and your body undergoes additional age-related changes. Although you might hear that it is usually best to start with the lowest dosages possible, this may not be true for younger women. Higher dosages may be prescribed in order to better compensate, and dosages will have to be reevaluated depending on how you are feeling and which symptoms are bothering you.

BENEFITS AND RISKS OF HT

There are many symptoms associated with estrogen deficiency, particularly vaginal dryness, hot flashes, and sleep disruption.* There are also more "hidden" changes that can have a huge impact later in life, such as osteoporosis and early heart disease. As a result, low estrogen levels can contribute to a bone fracture or even heart attack as you get older.

HT involving estrogens is very effective at reducing (and sometimes even completely preventing) the symptoms associated with low estrogen levels. Most women see an improvement in their symptoms within three to four weeks of starting HT. In terms of long-term health concerns, HT has been shown to improve bone density and prevent bone loss. Similarly, it may delay the onset of heart disease. However, more recent research has disputed this, stating that HT may not benefit the heart as much as once thought. Current research is focusing on whether HT can reduce the risk of other serious diseases, such as colon cancer and Alzheimer's.

There are several side effects associated with HT, including nausea, headaches, breast tenderness, increased blood pressure, and weight gain. If any of these side effects is experienced, you can change your HT regimen and see if the symptoms subside. Usually, the lower the dosage of the HT the fewer side effects are experienced. It is unclear whether younger women experience the same side effects in the same ways.

HT risk is related to:

- A woman's baseline disease risks
- Age
- Cause of ovarian insufficiency
- Time since symptoms began
- Prior use of any hormone
- HT types, routes of administration, and doses used
- Medical conditions emerging during treatment

* Women also regularly report skin issues and changes in mood.

For example, we have learned that there may be a higher risk of blood clots among women taking HT. These blood clots (called deep vein thromboses) occur in the leg veins. If you have experienced a blood clot before, HT should not be used. The risk of stroke might also be raised in women taking HT, so women who have had a history of coronary heart disease, blood clots, or strokes, or are at high risk for these complications, should discuss this with their health care provider.

Cancer is another major concern for women on HT. If progesterone is also taken, there does not seem to be any increased risk of uterine cancer. As for breast cancer, several studies have suggested that the risk of breast cancer may be higher in women who have taken HT for many years. If there is a strong family history of breast cancer (for instance, your mother and/or sister has had breast cancer), it is wise to talk to a specialist about your own risk.

WHAT'S BEST FOR ME?

While hormone therapy is an important issue for younger women experiencing ovarian insufficiency, always talk to your doctor about figuring out the best regimen. There is still a lot we don't know, so make sure you talk with your health care provider regularly about this topic.

Even though little research has been conducted that specifically looks at younger women and HT, it is possible that women who experience diminishing ovarian function have a lower-than-average risk for developing thrombosis and breast cancer. Replacing estrogen via HT would then return these risks to "normal," as if the ovaries were not becoming insufficient.

Since HT does not suppress your own hormone production, you may actually begin to experience more side effects, including heavier bleeding, while on HT, due to an excess of hormones. Some experts recommend that younger women on HT have regular testing to monitor the uterine lining and prevent any long-term problems. While HT is a complicated issue, most doctors believe that its benefits outweigh its risks for younger women with insufficient ovaries.

The following is a primer on which hormones are typically replaced.

ESTROGEN THERAPY

Estrogen therapy comes in a number of dosages and different forms: tablets, patches, gels, rings, and creams. Estrogen therapy provides the estrogen that the ovaries would normally produce and provides relief from the symptoms caused by low levels of estrogen.

HT can be continuous or cyclical. Continuous, or continuous combined, HT involves taking both estrogen and progestin or progesterone every day. Cyclical, or cyclical combined, usually involves taking estrogen every day of the month and progestin or progesterone for only part of each month. This is also sometimes referred to as sequential HT.

ORAL CONJUGATED EQUINE ESTROGENS Conjugated estrogens are extracted from the urine of pregnant horses and used to make tablets. Since they have been around the longest, these types of estrogen replacement are the most widely used type of estrogen. As a result, we have the most scientific data on the associated benefits and risks.

ORAL CONJUGATED EQUINE ESTROGENS

Brand Name	Manufacturer	Dosage Options
Premarin	Wyeth Pharmaceuticals	0.3, 0.45, 0.625 (standard), 0.9, 1.25 mg

OTHER ORAL ESTROGENS Other tablet medications are synthetic copies of the natural compounds extracted from plant sources. Similar in strength to the conjugated equine estrogens, they have not been around quite as long, so they lack the many years of scientific research investigating their benefits and risks. Still, they do seem to be as effective as the conjugated estrogens. There are three major types of oral estrogen medications: estradiol, esterified estrogen, and conjugated estrogen.

OTHER ORAL ESTROGENS

Brand Name	Type	Manufacturer	Dosage Options
Estrace	oral estradiol	Warner Chilcott	0.5, 1, 2 mg
Gynodiol	oral estradiol	Novavax	0.5, 1, 1.5, 2 mg
Menest	oral esterified estrogen	King Pharmaceuticals	0.3, 0.625, 1.25, 2.5 mg
Ogen	oral esterified estrogen	Pharmacia & Upjohn	0.625, 1.25, 2.5 mg estropipate
Enjuvia	conjugated estrogen	Duramed	0.3, 0.45, 0.625, 0.9, 1.25 mg

ESTROGEN SKIN PATCHES Skin patches allow estrogen to be slowly absorbed gradually through the skin (transdermally) directly into your bloodstream. Patches are applied directly to your skin below your waist, for example, on your thigh, buttock, hip, or stomach. The patches contain estradiol, a synthetic copy of an estrogen made by the ovary. They are changed periodically, from every few days to once a week. In general, many women experience fewer side effects with patches than with tablets. More specifically, estrogen patches are helpful in reducing headaches, nausea, and a rise in blood pressure. Additionally, patches are useful for women with liver disease or elevated cholesterol levels. Patches are preferred by many clinicians because they bypass the liver and do not increase clotting or triglycerides.

Since they are so easy to use and have so few side effects, many women, especially younger women, prefer patches over oral methods. One common side effect of patches is skin irritation. If this occurs, try to stick the patch on a different spot until the irritation clears up. It is also a good idea to vary where you stick it each time to minimize the chance of irritation. The dosage of estrogen patches varies from 0.025 to 0.1 mg of estradiol absorbed through the skin every 24 hours.

SKIN PATCHES

Brand Name	Manufacturer	Dosage Options
Estraderm	Novartis Pharmaceuticals	0.05, 0.1 mg
Climara	Bayer HealthCare Pharmaceuticals	0.025, 0.0375, 0.05, 0.06, 0.075, 0.1 mg
Vivelle and Vivelle-Dot	Novogyne Pharmaceuticals	0.025, 0.0375, 0.05, 0.075, 0.1 mg
Alora	Watson	0.025, 0.05, 0.075, 0.1 mg

HAVING TROUBLE GETTING YOUR PATCH TO STICK?

Make sure your hands and the area where you are going to put the patch are completely clean and free of any oils, lotions, and powders. Swab the area where you want to apply the patch with rubbing alcohol and allow it to dry completely. Apply the patch and hold it down with the palm of your hand for several seconds.

If the patch becomes loose or gets water under it, remove it, dry the area completely, and then reapply the patch. Hold it down with the palm of your hand, or try giving it a shot of warm air from a hair dryer.

If all this fails, talk to your health care provider about switching to another brand of patch that might stick to your skin better.

ESTROGEN GELS Estrogen gels work similarly to patches in that the estrogen is absorbed transdermally, or directly into the bloodstream through the skin. The gel can be applied to the arms, shoulders, or thighs every day.

ESTROGEN ESTRADIOL GELS

Brand Name	Manufacturer
EstroGel	Ascend Therapeutics
Elestrin	Azur Pharma

VAGINAL ESTROGEN There are several different forms of vaginal estrogen, including creams, tablets, and rings. These types of estrogen are prescribed to alleviate some of the symptoms of low estrogen levels, particularly those that affect sexual functioning, such as vaginal dryness and irritation. These medications work topically to replace hormone levels, and they usually take up to three to four weeks before you start noticing their effect.

Estrogen creams, such as Estrace and Premarin, are applied directly to the vagina every day. Depending on the dosage, a vaginal cream can deliver about the same amount of estrogen into the body as an oral method of estrogen replacement. In order to properly use an estrogen cream, wash your hands before using the cream. Fill the supplied applicator with the medicine according to the directions. Insert the applicator high into the vagina, and press the plunger to release the medication. Wash the applicator with warm, soapy water and rinse well after each use. Since the cream can sometimes be messy, it is best to apply it at bedtime, and you will probably want to wear a panty liner.

Vaginal tablet forms of estrogen replacement typically produce lower levels of estrogen than taking estrogen by mouth or skin patch. Vagifem is a vaginal estrogen tablet inserted into the vagina daily that offers an effective, clean, convenient, and comfortable treatment option. It is not recommended for women who have had certain types of uterine cancer.

A vaginal ring is a flexible plastic ring inserted into the vagina every three months. Once inserted, it remains in place and does not need to be removed even during intercourse or bathing. Most women (and their partners) say it cannot be felt. A vaginal ring may be preferred by women who have trouble remembering to apply a cream or take a tablet every day. Some vaginal rings provide a higher dosage of estrogen and may lead to more systemic effects, meaning that they may also influence symptoms beyond just vaginal dryness and irritation. The vaginal estrogen ring and the vaginal estrogen tablet release about one-tenth the dose of estrogen into the bloodstream than do oral or skin-patch estrogen replacement medicines.

I love the Estring. Seriously, the vaginal ring is easy to deal with, it can be left in place for three months and then a new one inserted. It has made a huge difference in the way my vaginal area feels. I intend to use the Estring as long as necessary to keep the area feeling healthy.

—Tori

In order to properly insert a vaginal ring, squeeze the sides of the ring together and insert it into the vagina as far as possible. You should not be able to feel the ring once it is in place. If you can still feel it, use a finger to push it in farther. Don't worry, it is not possible for the ring to go in too far or become lost. It can be left in place for up to ninety days. If it ever falls out, rinse it with warm water and reinsert it. It if slides down, just push it back up. After ninety days, remove the ring and re-place it with a new one. To remove the ring, just loop a finger though it and gently pull it from the vagina.

Vaginal Estrogen

Brand Name	Type	Manufacturer	Dosage Options
Estrace	cream (estradiol)	Warner Chilcott	0.1 mg estradiol/gram
Premarin	cream (conjugated estrogen)	Wyeth Pharmaceuticals	0.625 mg equine conjugated estrogen/ gram
Estring	vaginal ring	Pfizer	0.0075 mg estradiol per day released over three months
Femring	vaginal ring	Warner Chilcott	0.05 mg per day, 0.1 mg per day
Vagifem	vaginal tablet	Novo Nordisk Femcare	0.025 mg estradiol per tablet

What If You Forget a Dose?

If you forget an estrogen replacement dose, do it as soon as you remember. If it is close to the time of your next dose, skip the first one. Do not take two doses of estrogen in one day.

ESTROGEN EMULSIONS Estrogen emulsions, similar to a lotion, are also available. An emulsion can be applied to the legs each morning. Each foil-laminated pouch should be opened individually. Using your hands, rub the contents of one pouch into the entire thigh and calf of your left leg for about three minutes or until it is thoroughly absorbed. Open another pouch, and repeat the process for your right leg. Any excess can be rubbed into the buttocks. Allow the areas to dry completely before covering with clothes. Finally, wash your hands with soap and water to remove any residual medication.

ESTROGEN EMULSIONS

Brand Name	Type	Manufacturer
Estrasorb	Soy-based lotion	Graceway Pharmaceuticals
Evamist	Plant-based skin spray	Ther-Rx Corporation

PROGESTERONE THERAPY

For women who still have a uterus, it is important to have progesterone replacement therapy along with estrogen replacement therapy. One of progesterone's most important functions is to maintain the lining of the uterus, or endometrium. Without progesterone, the lining cannot be regularly shed and tends to build up. This condition increases the risk of certain types of cancers affecting the uterus and endometrium.

There are a number of medications that help counteract low levels of progesterone in the body. Progestins, the most common form, are synthetic versions of progesterone. Progestins have been around since the 1950s and are very close to the body's own natural progesterone. However, because they are slightly different from natural progesterone, they sometimes cause side effects such as headaches, breast tenderness, weight gain, and moodiness. Since each progestin is formulated slightly differently, it is difficult to generalize the side effects. Provera is the most commonly prescribed progestin by far and is also available in a generic form called medroxyprogesterone acetate, which costs significantly less. It is typically taken as either a 5 mg or 10 mg dose for five to fourteen days a month. Bleeding usually occurs about three to seven days after you stop taking it.

Originally, synthetic progesterones were developed because they could be absorbed into the bloodstream more easily. Recently, it has been found that micronization of progesterone (making very tiny crystals of the progesterone) enhances absorption from the gastrointestinal tract. As a result, micronized progesterone is sometimes used instead of progestins. Many patients report that natural progesterones do not seem to have as many side effects. The most commonly prescribed natural progesterone is Prometrium, an oral micronized capsule.

> **WARNING!**
> Some brands of progesterone capsules contain peanut oil and may trigger a life-threatening allergic reaction in people who are allergic to peanuts.

Although there are several nonprescription progesterone creams on the market, the necessary dosage needed to protect the uterus is unknown. Thus, it is not recommended that women depend on this method of progesterone supplementation.

ESTROGEN AND PROGESTERONE COMBINATIONS

Since women with diminishing ovarian function still have an intact uterus and are probably still getting their periods occasionally, it is important that HT for them include both estrogen and progesterone. To make things easier, there are several different products that include both types of medication. There is really no difference between taking these combination pills and taking two separate similar estrogen and progestin tablets. Of course, it is also much easier to remember to take one medication than two. The side effects are the same, but you will need to talk to your health care provider about your individual risks based on your specific medical history.

Prempro and Premphase are the most commonly prescribed combination pills for younger women. The standard dosage is 0.625 mg of conjugated estrogen and 2.5 mg of medroxyprogesterone acetate (progestin). Prempro is taken every day; with Premphase, you take the progestin for only two weeks out of the month. Other common dosages include 0.3 mg estrogen/1.5 mg of medroxyprogesterone acetate; 0.45 mg estrogen/1.5 mg medroxyprogesterone acetate; and 0.625 mg estrogen/5 mg medroxyprogesterone acetate.

BIRTH CONTROL PILLS

Since birth control pills contain hormones, many women ask about the difference between HT and birth control pills. Though birth control pills are most often given as a form of contraception, women who are experiencing POI, early menopause, or perimenopause are sometimes prescribed them to boost their hormone levels, and minimize symptoms especially if they are still getting periods. Unfortunately, it is common for women to be given a prescription before any testing is conducted and they are accurately diagnosed. As a result, symptoms are masked and a proper diagnosis is even further delayed. Ovarian insufficiency goes beyond just fertility and includes many other serious health-related concerns.

A proper diagnosis is imperative before starting any type of HT, including birth control pills. In order to prevent long-term consequences of low hormone levels, such as osteoporosis, hormone therapy needs to be at the appropriate dosage.

Birth control pills contain both a synthetic estrogen and progestin, in different dosage combinations depending on the specific brand. Ethinyl estradiol is a strong synthetic estrogen contained in birth control pills that inhibits ovulation. However, because synthetic estrogens are more powerful than natural estrogens (roughly four to ten times as strong), they may contribute to a higher risk of blood clotting than other forms of HT. This risk increases even more if you are over thirty-five years old and if you smoke, which is why birth control pills are not recommended for women in those groups.

Another downside is that with oral contraceptives, estrogen is provided for only three of every four weeks, the fourth week being hormone free. For women who are already estrogen deficient, the lack of estrogen in this week may cause symptoms to return or worsen. Consequently, it may be more helpful to consider continuous estrogen through other forms of HT. Though many believe birth control pills are more socially acceptable for younger women than HT, they are not as effective in preventing long-term health concerns.

TESTOSTERONE REPLACEMENT

Since the ovary makes about half of the supply of testosterone in women, low testosterone levels are common among women with diminishing ovarian function. Some women find that the lower levels of testosterone reduce sex drive and energy. To counteract this, testosterone supplementation is available in either tablet or implant form. However, it can result in many side effects, including excess hair growth, especially on the face; acne; and increased cholesterol levels. For this reason, testosterone treatment is not given routinely. The overall benefits and risks of testosterone therapy have not been established by the FDA, so you should discuss your own needs and concerns with your health care provider.

Some physicians instead prescribe a testosterone precursor called dehydroepiandrosterone (DHEA), which seems to provide a slight boost to low testosterone levels without as many side effects. Still, there are little data available about the long-term effects of DHEA, especially among women. Evidence suggests that increased levels of male hormones may increase the risk of certain hormone-sensitive cancers, such as breast and ovarian cancer. Therefore, testosterone supplementation is not recommended for regular use without careful supervision by a trained health care professional.

In general, testosterone treatment should be considered only for women who have had their ovaries removed or who clearly suffer from severely diminishing ovarian function, who are taking an effective hormone regimen, and who are still having problems. Even in those cases, they should take only the lowest dose of testosterone available.

How to Adjust Your HT Regimen

Starting HT made me very moody and depressed. My doctor didn't believe me, said, "Now you know how all women feel." If that was true, all women would have already ripped off all the heads of all the men. I was a terror on them consistently, with no ups and downs. Finally, after I changed doctors, I changed dosages and life is better for everyone. I've gone in for hormone therapy adjustments half a dozen times so far, and I probably will again. I have gotten my medications adjusted for breakthrough bleeding, hot flushes, depression, cramps in my legs, complete lack of libido, and a skin reaction to certain patches.

—Brooke

An effective health care provider makes adjustments to your hormones based on whether your symptoms are relieved. The dose, form, and regimen of the medications are determined depending on your individual background, current symptoms, family history, medical history, and goals for the hormone therapy. It's time to talk to your health care provider about adjusting your HT if your symptoms change for the worse, if you experience breakthrough bleeding, or you have a reaction to a certain medication. Another reason for an adjustment may be that the current medication and dosage just don't work the way you had hoped they would and you want to try a different approach.

THE ART OF HORMONE THERAPY

Your doctor should be able to tailor your HT to meet your needs and how you are feeling. For some women, it can take several months or even up to a year to find the appropriate dosages. You should definitely keep the lines of communication open at all times and talk with your doctor honestly about how you are feeling and if you are experiencing any side effects. Remember that HT is a process, and your specific dosage and regimen may change as you age or other aspects of your life change.

HT Research and You

Over the last several years, much attention has rightfully been paid to results from the Women's Health Initiative, a study of hormone therapy for postmenopausal women, mostly in their fifties or older. In fact, the average age was sixty-three. The study concluded that while hormone therapy protected against bone loss, it slightly increased the risk of developing breast cancer and heart disease. However, before you apply these findings to your decision making about hormone therapy, it is important to know that the women in this study who took hormone therapy were very different from young women who experience diminishing ovarian function.

For younger women, the ovaries "should" have continued to make the hormones estrogen and progesterone for many more years, as the natural age of menopause is typically around fifty-one. Hormone therapy for younger women is much closer to true "replacement" of what the ovaries should be making while they are in their thirties and forties.

In contrast, women who participated in the Women's Health Initiative were taking hormone therapy past the time nature intended for the ovaries to be making hormones. They were in effect extending their lifetime exposure to hormones beyond what nature intended. POI researcher Dr. Lawrence Nelson explains, "It is important that our patients realize that the recent report is a study about menopausal women, not young women with ovarian insufficiency. As we have been emphasizing to our patients for years, it is important to remember that premature ovarian failure is not a premature menopause. There are many important ways that premature ovarian failure differs from the normal menopause. It is not scientifically valid to make conclusions about young women with premature ovarian failure based on findings in older women with menopause. In the recent report older women with menopause extended their exposure to hormones for years beyond what nature intended.

"Also, the hormone regimen in the report was completely different from what we recommend to our patients. The estrogen used in the study was horse estrogen, and we recommend using the natural human estrogen called estradiol. Also, the estrogen in the study was given by mouth, which might have contributed to the increased cardiovascular risk.

"For years we have been recommending use of the estradiol patch. We have recommended this because the estradiol patch avoids the first-pass effect on the liver and provides estradiol in a more natural manner, similar to how the ovary works. The patch provides estradiol a little bit at a time in a constant manner into the veins rather than one big dose in a pill once a day; when taken by mouth it has to get past the liver before entering the blood, which can cause problems. Also, the post-menopausal women who participated in the recently reported study took the progestin every day. We typically recommend taking it only twelve days each month."

Stopping HT

You may decide to stop using HT for a number of reasons. If you need to have additional medical tests, for example, you will need to be off HT for several weeks beforehand. You may decide you no longer want to take HT and wish to see if you can manage the symptoms and long-term risks with other approaches. Or you may need to go off before beginning fertility treatment. Whatever the reason, stopping "cold turkey" may not be the best approach. Some health care providers recommend taking half of the treatment dosages for one month, others recommend a longer-term approach to minimize symptoms. Always talk to your health care provider, and create a plan.

Deciding Against HT

I was told numerous things about starting or not starting HT by each doctor I met with—obviously with each contradicting the other. For now, I decided against taking HT. That's the right decision for me at this time. It may change; it probably will change down the road. The long-term health and impact on my bones are something that concerns me, but the steps I am taking toward this are taking calcium tablets every day, converting to soya milk, and weight training.

—Moira

For some women, the perceived risks of HT may be too great, or a health condition may preclude HT as a viable treatment. In any case, make sure the decision you make is an informed one. Do your homework. One of the most important things you can do is be honest with your health care provider. He or she thinks you should be on hormone therapy, and you don't want to be, at least for now. Many women decide to accept the prescription so their doctor will be quiet, then either never fill it or don't get refills when it runs out. In fact, in one large study, researchers found that one year after the initial prescription of hormone therapy, 54.4 percent of the study subjects were noncompliant. The biggest factor in compliance? The age of the patient. The younger the woman, the less likely she was to take her HT as recommended, if at all.

If you are going to stand your ground and refuse HT, be honest with your health care provider. Brainstorm together to find alternate ways to address concerns about your health. One compromise might be to have a bone scan done to determine the health of your bones. The results may help you make an informed decision about your osteoporosis risks, for example. Don't waste your time, energy, and resources—or your health care provider's knowledge—without a frank discussion about what you are willing to do (or not do) in your situation.

10

Complementary and Lifestyle Treatments

I think just knowing that there is a problem throws our bodies out even more because we have ongoing worries and heartache, which has never been good for anyone's cycle. Just to give you a little hope, my periods stopped for over a whole year and I have been told countless times that this means full-blown menopause, to get some HT, and one doc told me to get my head out of the sand and face it. I've never been one to conform to the norm, so eventually after various routes I went and got a supplement and good food plan from a nutritionist, moved house to a very peaceful area, and do more things that make me happy. And guess what? My periods have returned. That's without HT too. They are doctors, not gods. And I'm not inclined to believe what they predict about my body when they can't even tell me why this has happened in the first place. They only know what they have been taught, and they're all singing from the same hymn sheet.

—Sharon

MANY WOMEN EXPERIENCING PREMATURE ovarian insufficiency use complementary and alternative medicine (CAM). According to the National Institutes of Health (NIH), complementary and alternative medicine is a group of diverse medical and health care systems, practices, and products that are not generally considered part of conventional medicine. Generally, complementary medicine is used together with standard medical care. An example is using acupuncture to help with side effects of cancer treatment.

The world of complementary medicine is a logical avenue to consider when our view of health has been thrown into such turmoil, explains the reproductive counselor Karin A. Clark, director of the Center for Conceiving Health. "The medical world," she says, "has dished out an untenable decree about our lives, and we feel helpless and let down. Nothing can be done in that world to make this better, no one can give us an answer to 'why' other than the small percentage of women who fall into the 'genetic' category. We want help. We need hope. For some of us the hope we seek is for peace, health, resolution. For others, the desire for a miracle is our real pursuit.

"Practitioners of more holistic modalities, whether naturopathy, herbalism, counseling, acupuncture—or some combination of all of them—can offer hope for balance, greater vitality, relief from depression and anxiety, and the opening of a world of new ideas and tools to enhance our lives going forward. We lose the benefits of all of these when we look at any of the people or modalities we seek out as our savior or the magic person to make this 'all better.' Don't get me wrong! I do believe in miracles. I do believe the body is capable of remarkable things. I also believe that the magic is in us and we lose the power of that potential whenever we believe someone else can heal us. Others can give us tools and guidance to help us move into our dreams, even if we have been forced to craft new ones."

> *There are five main types of CAM:*
> - Biologically based therapies, such as herbal and botanical supplements
> - Alternative medical systems, such as traditional Chinese medicine
> - Mind-body interventions, such as biofeedback and hypnosis
> - Manipulative and body-based methods, such as massage therapy
> - Energy therapies, such as Reiki

Karin A. Clark explains that you have likely had the help of a team to reach your diagnosis, and continuing to build an effective team from a broad variety of disciplines is important. "It is the reflection of wisdom to build a team to move you forward from here. The world of complementary medicine offers great potential for a lifetime of supportive, healing people to nurture and nourish you as you move into the new life story that you will be creating now."

Though we are very supportive of complementary therapies in a number of health situations, they are not appropriate for everyone. The following are some of the major kinds.

Biologically Based Therapies

This is the area of complementary care that draws the most attention on message boards, in doctor's offices, and among support groups of women undergoing POI or other forms of diminishing ovarian function. After all, Oprah Winfrey, Robin McGraw (Dr. Phil's wife), and Suzanne Somers have generated tons of attention focusing on this issue, so these therapies must be great, right? Maybe not.

BIOIDENTICAL HORMONES

There's a lot of interest in bioidentical—so-called natural—hormone therapy for menopause symptoms. Bioidentical hormones are custommixed formulas containing various hormones that are chemically identical to those naturally made by your body. These prescription and over-the-counter products are marketed as being tailored to a woman's individual hormone needs, typically determined through saliva hormone testing. Ever since Suzanne Somers published *The Sexy Years*, women have been clamoring for information on bioidentical hormones. If they could relieve Suzanne Somers's menopausal symptoms and breathe fire back into her lagging sex life, what could they do for us mere mortals? The truth is—who knows? There is far too little evidence available to make an informed decision in favor of bioidentical hormones at this time.

The terms *bioidentical, natural,* and *compounded* sex hormones started to gain visibility in the media a few years ago. Despite its outwardly "scientific" appearance, the term "bioidentical hormones" is quite vague and is used in various contexts. There are no bioidentical hormones that do not undergo some sort of laboratory manipulation. Consequently, there are no truly "natural" bioidentical hormones.

Most commonly, this term denotes plant-derived hormones that are claimed to be "identical in structure" to those produced by the human body. The "bioidentical" approach generally also refers to the use of an individualized dose of hormones that is made by a compounding pharmacy as pills, creams, or vaginal suppositories. The quality of these products is not regulated and in many cases is inferior to prescription medications.

The hormones that are most commonly included in these bioidentical formulas are estradiol, estrone, estriol, progesterone, testosterone, and DHEA. A woman is typically asked to provide a saliva or blood sample, which is used to measure her baseline hormone levels. Based on these results, the prescriber selects the individual hormones and the doses to be compounded.

There is no evidence that these hormones have any advantage over conventional HT, and their safety has not been established. Moreover, they have not been studied with respect to their effect on long-term effects of diminishing hormones levels that specifically affect younger women.

The term "bioidentical" is really confusing. In fact, "bioidentical" is not a scientific term and is used by different people to mean different things. Dr. Valerie Baker explains, "I would like to think of it as meaning closest to the natural forms and doses of estradiol and progesterone that the ovary makes, and in principle I think that that is a good goal with hormone therapy. In common use, however, the term 'biochemical' is used to mean that the hormone is plant-derived or from natural sources or not marketed by a pharmaceutical company (and often not regulated), rather than synthesized in a lab, and in this way it is often used as a marketing tool. Sometimes, what is marketed as being most natural isn't really the closest to what the ovary makes."

INCONSISTENCY IS AN ISSUE Bioidentical hormones are often custom-compounded, containing one or more of various hormones in differing amounts, depending on an individual prescriber's order. The recipe contains not only the active hormone (or hormones) but also other ingredients that either hold everything together (in the case of a rectal suppository, an under-the-tongue tablet, or an under-the-skin pellet) or provides a vehicle for applying the product onto the skin (such as a cream or gel) or into the body (such as a liquid for a nasal spray).

These compounds do not have government approval because individually mixed recipes have not been tested to prove that they are absorbed appropriately or provide predictable levels in blood and tissue. And, according to a statement from the North American Menopause Society, which has expressed concern regarding bioidentical hormones,

> there is no scientific evidence about the effects of these hormones on the body, both good and bad. Preparation methods vary from one pharmacist to another, and from one pharmacy to another, which means that patients may not receive consistent amounts of medication. In addition, inactive ingredients may vary and there can be batch-to-batch differences. Reliable sterility and freedom from undesired contaminants are also concerns. In fact, the FDA analyzed a variety of twenty-nine product samples from twelve compounding pharmacies and found that 34 percent of them failed one or more standard quality tests.

BIOIDENTICAL HORMONE REPLACEMENT THERAPY (BHRT) SIDE EFFECTS

If bioidentical products were unsafe, there would be a lot of reports of bad side effects, right? Not so, says the FDA. "Unlike commercial drug manufacturers, pharmacies aren't required to report adverse events associated with compounded drugs," says Steve Silverman, the assistant director of the Office of Compliance of the FDA's Center for Drug Evaluation and Research. "Also, while some health risks associated with 'BHRT' drug products may arise after a relatively short period of use, others may not occur for many years. One of the big problems is that we just don't know what risks are associated with these so-called bioidenticals. Expense is also an issue, as many custom-compounded preparations are viewed as experimental drugs and are not covered by insurance plans."

FINDING A PROVIDER

If you choose to further investigate bioidentical hormone replacement therapy, ask your health care provider these questions:

- How long have you been working with BHRT?
- Are you a board-certified physician (in endocrinology, internal medicine, gynecology, etc.)?

- How often have you worked with women with my specific condition?
- Are hormone levels being measured by blood work or a hair or saliva test? (Blood tests are the proven way to get the best results.)

WHAT DOES "BOARD-CERTIFIED" MEAN?

Being board-certified in medicine means a physician has taken and passed a medical specialty examination. Board-eligible, by contrast, means that a physician has completed the requirements for admission to a medical specialty board examination but has not taken and passed the examination. For example, a physician must do three years of training in an approved pediatric residency to be board-eligible and then successfully complete a comprehensive written examination to be certified by the American Board of Pediatrics. Go to www.certifieddoctor.org to verify a physician's credentials in the American Board of Medical Specialties (ABMS).

PURCHASING BIOIDENTICAL HORMONES

If you choose to take BHRT, allow a trained pharmacist to compound the appropriate prescription. It is much more likely that the hormones used will have been tested for purity and concentration. If the medication is purchased from an Internet site, you are less likely to know what you are getting.

In order to locate a compounding pharmacist near you, check with the Professional Compounding Centers of American (PCCA) at www.pccarx.com or 800-331-2498.

PHYTOESTROGENS

Some botanical products, such as soy and red clover, contain weak estrogenlike compounds called phytoestrogens. Some women eat specific foods that contain phytoestrogens to get their estrogenic effects. The food most commonly known to contain phytoestrogens is soy, but beans, peas, lentils, and whole grains and seeds, especially flaxseed, rye, and millet, also contain them.

Alternatives like these are much less likely to be studied in formal research trials than drugs are, but there are some data from both observational and randomized controlled trials. Some studies have shown that eating foods containing phytoestrogens provides modest relief of hot flashes, while other studies have found that eating foods containing phytoestrogens causes changes in vaginal cells that are similar to the changes caused by taking estrogen and could relieve discomfort.

However, it is uncertain whether this relief comes from phytoestrogens or from other compounds in the plants. Much remains to be learned about these plant products, including exactly how they work in the human body. Health care providers caution that certain women need to be particularly careful about using phytoestrogens, especially:

- Women who have had or are at increased risk of diseases or conditions that are affected by hormones, such as breast, uterine, or ovarian cancer; endometriosis; or uterine fibroids
- Women who are taking drugs that increase estrogen levels in the body, such as birth control pills or a type of cancer drug called a selective estrogen receptor modulator (SERM), such as tamoxifen

NUTRITIONAL SUPPLEMENTS

As mentioned above, natural remedies are biologically active substances and need to be respected every bit as much as prescription meds. Almost any drug we use originally comes from herbs or plants. There are some herbs that are known to have beneficial therapeutic effects, such as soy for relieving menopausal symptoms and ginger to prevent nausea and vomiting. However, there are currently no drugs or herbs known to induce ovulation in the patient with diminishing ovarian function. You also have to keep in mind that until we test an herb by grinding it up, measuring it out, and testing it in a placebo-controlled trial, we don't know for sure what the active ingredient in an herbal remedy is or if it really works.

The National Center for Complementary and Alternative Medicine (NCCAM) emphasizes the importance of speaking with your health care provider about any complementary and alternative practices you use, including dietary supplements. Give your clinician a complete picture of what you do to manage your health. This will help ensure coordinated and safe care. It is especially important to talk to your health care provider if you are:

- Thinking about replacing your regular medication with one or more dietary supplements
- Taking any medications (whether prescription or over the counter), as some dietary supplements have been found to interact with medications
- Planning to have surgery; certain dietary supplements may increase the risk of bleeding or affect your response to anesthesia
- Pregnant or nursing a baby or considering giving a child a dietary supplement; most dietary supplements have not been tested in pregnant women, nursing mothers, or children

(For more information about talking with your health care providers about CAM, see NCCAM's Time to Talk campaign at nccam.nih.gov/ timetotalk.)

Alternative Medical Systems

Alternative medical systems have evolved apart from and often earlier than the conventional medical approach used in the United States. Examples of medical systems that have developed in Western cultures include homeopathic medicine and naturopathic medicine. Examples of systems that have developed in non-Western cultures include traditional Chinese medicine (TCM) and Ayurveda.

Though scientific evidence exists regarding some CAM therapies, for most there are key questions that are yet to be answered through well-designed scientific studies, such as whether these therapies are safe and effective as well as whether they work for the purposes for which they are used.

AYURVEDA

According to the Ayurvedic Institute, Ayurveda is the ancient art of healing that has been practiced continuously for more than five thousand years. The principles of many natural healing systems now familiar in the West, such as homeopathy and polarity therapy, have their roots in Ayurveda. Ayurvedic practices, it is claimed, restore the balance and harmony of the individual, resulting in self-healing, good health, and increased longevity.

Ayurvedic medicine is defined by the National Center for Alternative and Complementary Medicine as an attempt to "integrate and balance the body, mind, and spirit; thus, some view it as 'holistic.' This balance is believed to lead to happiness and health, and to help prevent illness. Ayurvedic medicine also treats specific physical and mental health problems. A chief aim of Ayurvedic practices is to cleanse the body of substances that can cause disease, thus helping to reestablish harmony and balance."

TRADITIONAL CHINESE MEDICINE

In traditional Chinese medicine (TCM), the understanding of the human body is based on the holistic theory of the universe as described in Daoism, and the treatment of illness is based primarily on the diagnosis and differentiation of syndromes. Acupuncture is the practice that most often comes to mind when thinking of Chinese medicine, but TCM is a much broader system of medicine that includes herbs, massage, diet, and exercise therapy. The underlying theory is that all of creation is born from the interdependence of two opposite principles, yin and yang. These two opposites are in constant motion, creating a fluctuating balance in the healthy body. Disease results when either yin or yang is in a state of prolonged excess or deficiency.

CHOOSING A CAM PRACTITIONER

When you choose any type of CAM practitioner, you will want to be well prepared for your first visit. Here are some suggested questions to ask a new provider:

- What benefits can I expect from this therapy?
- What are the risks associated with this therapy?
- Do the benefits outweigh the risks for my disease or condition?
- What side effects can be expected?
- Will the therapy interfere with any of my daily activities?
- How long will I need to undergo treatment? How often will my progress or plan of treatment be assessed?

- Will I need to buy any equipment or supplies?
- Do you have scientific articles or references about using the treatment for my condition?
- Could the therapy interact with conventional treatments?
- Are there any conditions for which this treatment should not be used?

Mind-Body Interventions

Mind-body interventions use a variety of techniques designed to enhance the mind's capacity to affect bodily function and symptoms. Some techniques that were considered to be CAM in the past (for example, patient support groups and cognitive behavioral therapy) have become mainstream. Other mind-body techniques are still considered CAM, including meditation, prayer, mental healing, and therapies that use creative outlets such as art, music, or dance.

"Our body has let us down, or so we think. We feel betrayed by it, perhaps. Betrayed by life even. And yet to feel better," explains Karin A. Clark, "to have life return to something we can love and look forward to, we are faced with the daunting task of loving our body again, believing in our body again, and having the communication between our heart, our mind and our body deepen and grow. When we first receive the hard-hitting news like finding out our ovaries are not functioning properly, that possibility not only seems impossible, but undesirable. And yet that is where our hope and future joy lie, in that mind and body connection."

HYPNOTHERAPY

The hypnotherapy was done with a clinical hypnotherapist. My husband was very skeptical about it, but when he came along to some of the sessions, he knew it was doing some good. The hypnotherapist was helping with my self-esteem and general anxieties as I was suffering from depression at the time. He never told me that he would be able to help me get pregnant but he wanted to help me to relax and feel calmer about life, etc. I was knackered after each session, but he dug deep into my subconscious and somehow made me feel more relaxed with everyday life.

—Joylin

A new Baylor University study shows that hypnotic relaxation therapy can decrease the frequency and severity of hot flashes in menopausal women. "This study validates that this type of treatment is effective in decreasing hot flashes," says Dr. Gary Elkins, a professor of psychology and neuroscience at Baylor and a lead investigator on the project, which was published in the *Journal of Clinical Oncology.* "There is a real need to study emerging mind-body interactions to treating these ailments because there are times medications are not an option."

INFORMATION, PLEASE!

Want to find out more about complementary medicine but aren't sure where to start? The National Center for Complementary and Alternative Medicine (NCCAM) is the lead federal agency for complementary and alternative medicine (CAM) research and a component of the National Institutes of Health (NIH). Go to http://nccam.nih.gov.

"As we learn to listen to and honor our body," says Clark, "we will be stunned by our own inherent wisdom. The connection between our mind and body will become a rich and trusted ally on our path. As we relax our mind, we find our body responding with greater ease and comfort. As we stretch our bodies and move them toward great health, we find our minds becoming clearer and more flexible as well. The fissure that has separated the mind and body in our perception recedes, and with it, our sense of ourselves as whole, complete women can take root and blossom as well."

Manipulative and Body-Based Methods

Manipulative and body-based practices in CAM are based on manipulation, or the application of controlled force to a joint, moving it beyond the normal range of motion in an effort to aid in restoring health. Manipulation may be performed as a part of other therapies or medical systems, including chiropractic medicine, massage, and naturopathy.

NATUROPATHY

Naturopathic medicine is based on the belief that the human body has an innate healing ability. Naturopathic doctors (NDs) teach their patients to use diet, exercise, lifestyle changes, and cutting-edge natural therapies to enhance their bodies' ability to ward off and combat disease. According to the American Association of Naturopathic Physicians, "naturopathic physicians craft comprehensive treatment plans that blend the best of modern medical science and traditional natural medical approaches to not only treat disease, but to also restore health."

Energy Therapies

Energy therapies are intended to affect the energy fields that purportedly surround and penetrate the human body. The existence of such fields has not yet been scientifically proven. Some forms of energy therapy manipulate biofields by applying pressure and/or manipulating the body by placing the hands in, or through, these fields. Examples include Reiki and qi gong.

REIKI

Reiki is a Japanese technique of stress reduction and relaxation that also promotes healing. It is administered by "laying on hands" and is based on the idea that an unseen "life force energy" flows through us and is what causes us to be alive. If one's life force energy is low, we are more likely to get sick or feel stress, and if it is high, we are more capable of being happy and healthy, explains the International Center for Reiki Training. "The word Reiki is made of two Japanese words—Rei which means 'God's Wisdom or the Higher Power' and Ki which is 'life force energy.' So Reiki is actually 'spiritually guided life force energy.'"

QI GONG

Qi gong is a meditative movement exercise that reduces stress, improves blood flow to the internal organs, and exercises the body. "It is done in China and some modern Western clinics for healing, overcoming disease processes, and longevity. It is very good for fertility," explains Randine Lewis, Ph.D., a mind-body specialist licensed acupuncturist and herbalist.

Lifestyle Changes

Regardless of how you feel about these forms of alternative therapy, almost everyone can make some lifestyle choices to improve her health. Whether it's giving up a bad habit, such as smoking, or picking up a good one, such as exercising, take a critical look at your lifestyle and see what you can do to feel better.

DIET AND NUTRITION

If you are coping with shifting hormone levels, you may find that it's more difficult to lose extra pounds. Even if you always used to be able to eat whatever you liked and, even without exercise, were able to maintain your figure, that may change. Researchers suggest that weight gain occurs because of excessive ratios of progesterone to estradiol, which affects the rate of gastric emptying. In other words, explains Larrian Gillespie, M.D., author of *The Menopause Diet,* "we retain food longer in our stomachs and are more efficient at sucking out carbohydrates and storing them as fat." The result: the dreaded Buddha belly.

Gillespie suggests that women follow a diet that emphasizes foods low on the glycemic index—which means more protein, moderate amounts of good higher-fiber carbohydrates, and low saturated fats—to help with hormonal production. She's not alone in recommending a low-glycemic regimen. The American Diabetes Association began recommending it after research showed that dieters who followed a low-GI diet reduced inflammation markers significantly. The foods in a low-GI diet do not raise your blood sugar levels too high or too quickly. The diet itself is 40 percent protein, 25 percent fat, and 35 percent low-glycemic carbs.

"Good foods to include are dairy, full fat because of the requirement of vitamin D absorption, lots of vegetables, lean protein, and eggs. Make sure the eggs are never cooked hard because soft is ideal for absorption and minimal effect on cholesterol. Eat in-season foods for a wide variety of vitamins and nutrients. Never skip breakfast, and eat five smaller meals a day. Saturated fat in meats and other animal products are unhealthy for everyone. So reduce your intake of animal foods and choose lean meats."

Other foods Gillespie recommends include:

- Fruits such as melons and citrus are highly recommended; they are high in potassium and balance sodium and water retention.
- Dried fruit like apricots and figs.
- Vegetables, including yams, collard greens, and broccoli.
- Soy products, seaweed, and oily fish like tuna and salmon are some other beneficial foods.

EXERCISE

We all know that exercise is good for us. What else can we do that reduces our risk of developing cardiovascular disease and noninsulin dependent diabetes; helps us sleep; relieves stress; and increases energy, confidence, camaraderie, pride, relaxation, and sense of achievement? The same basic guidelines are true for all women. We should get thirty minutes of moderate-intensity physical activity on most days and preferably every day. Consider taking up a new activity that you may not have tried:

- Martial arts
- Belly dancing
- Salsa or other dance classes
- Swimming
- Cycling
- Yoga
- Team sports

Look for ways to increase your activity level daily. Examples include taking the stairs rather than the elevator, parking farther away from your destination, and buying (and using) a pedometer, aiming for 10,000 steps a day.

Some researchers believe there are specific exercise guidelines for women with lower ovarian function. Randine Lewis, Ph.D., the founder of Eastern Harmony Clinic, treats female infertility and recurrent miscarriage with traditional Chinese medicine. As an acupuncturist and herbalist, she explains, "I do not suggest sit-ups, Pilates, or any exercise that compresses the abdominal muscles. I like low-intensity exercises like walking, biking, and swimming. Yet if you are already in a regimen that is higher in intensity, I say do not exercise to the point of exhaustion or lift weights which require grunting to lift. We tend to exercise like men and divert our blood flow to the musculoskeletal system. Women are supposed to have rounder bellies that have room for growth, and are supposed to have a lot of blood going to the ovaries and uterus, not to the muscles. I highly recommend qi gong, tai chi, and yoga."

One of the best reasons to exercise is that it is thought to have a positive effect on mood. During exercise, hormones called endorphins are released in the brain. They are "feel good" hormones involved in the body's positive response to stress. The mood-heightening effect can last for several hours, according to some endocrinologists. Regular exercise benefits the heart and bones, helps regulate weight, and contributes to a sense of overall well-being and improvement in mood.

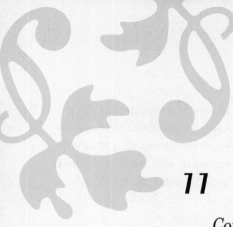

11

Coping with the Emotional and Physical Effects

After the initial shock of a diagnosis, there are two ways people can go about living with a medical disorder. They can be shy, ignore it, and beat themselves up for having a medical condition they cannot control. Or, they can accept themselves for who they are interpersonally as well as biologically and look beyond the stigma of having a medical disorder. I have chosen to live in the latter mode, and in doing so I have received an overwhelmingly positive response from doctors, researchers, family, friends, and the community. I have found that the more information people know about a medical disorder, the less scary it becomes and the more support they offer. Plus, I can focus more on adapting to my body's changes without focusing on what I've lost.

—Ellie

AS WE HAVE MENTIONED BEFORE, anytime your hormones are out of sync, other changes—both emotional and physical—are sure to follow. While getting appropriate medical care is an important component of effectively managing your condition, there is a lot you can do for yourself at home. Because you will spend much more time away from your doctor than with him or her, you will need to be an active member of your health care team if you are going to successfully manage your ovarian insufficiency and all your symptoms. Let's talk more about specific tools and techniques that will help you be successful in coping with all the emotional and physical effects of ovarian insufficiency.

Emotional Changes

Though wild mood swings may happen to lots of women, that doesn't mean you are powerless to address them. Consider some of the tools we suggest, but include your health care provider in the discussion as well. Because sleep deprivation and night sweats are also associated with moodiness, follow our recommendation to get a good night's sleep.

RELAX

We know it sounds cheesy, but relaxing helps. We know it isn't that easy. However, recent reports indicate that women who lead stressful lifestyles can suffer up to five times as many hot flashes as relaxed women. Your ability to cope with stress emotionally will affect how you feel physically. Massage, floating in water (a swimming pool or hot tub) or taking a relaxing bath, listening to a relaxation tape, doing slow deep breathing for several minutes, and yoga are all ways to help you find inner stillness and a quiet, peaceful mind.

The Mayo Clinic recommends that you practice a specific form of relaxation known as "paced respiration." Deep, slow abdominal breathing, known as paced respiration, can decrease hot flashes. It takes some practice to perfect the technique, but paced respiration done twice daily or at the beginning of a hot flash can be quite helpful. To practice paced respiration:

- Begin by sitting comfortably.
- Breathe in deeply for five seconds, pushing your stomach muscles out.
- Exhale for five seconds, pulling your stomach muscles in and up.
- Repeat this cycle of breathing deeply in and out until you feel calm and relaxed, either at the beginning of a hot flash or for fifteen minutes twice a day.

HOW TO IMPROVE YOUR MEMORY

You could tell me a phone number, and I would forget it midway through dialing, or I could be completing an application for a client, ask the zip code for their address, and two questions later have to enter the zip again and have to ask them to repeat it. Am I going crazy, or is this related to my hormones?

—Susan

It's possible that ovarian insufficiency can cause memory problems. Surgically induced menopause is associated with immediate decrements in estrogen levels as well as changes in cognition, specifically involving verbal memory. Or you could be experiencing "chemo fog" or insomnia. No one really knows, but there does appear to be some anecdotal connection between ovarian insufficiency and memory issues.

One research study suggested that the issue is not really impaired memory. Instead, they found a link between complaints of forgetfulness and the way stressed women learn or "encode" new information. "This is not what most people think of traditionally when they think of memory loss," said researcher Dr. Mark Mapstone, an assistant professor of neurology. "It feels like a memory problem, but the cause is different. It feels like you can't remember, but that's because you never really learned the information in the first place."

Mapstone likens the problem of encoding new information to a situation in which a doctor tells a patient that something serious may be wrong and gives a lot of detail. Afterward, she gets home and can hardly remember what the doctor said. It's not that she necessarily forgot what was said; it's more likely that she never really heard the doctor the first time because she was so anxious and worried. The same may be true of women with any hormone imbalance, many of whom live a life filled with stress and worry. Indeed, Mapstone also found that most of the women in the study had some sort of mood distress, including symptoms of depression or anxiety.

"When people spread their attention thin, it's difficult to encode new information. When they're worried or anxious about being late for work or the problems of an aging parent, that sort of stress can rob your attentional resources and impact your ability to encode information properly." Mapstone also said that difficulty taking in new information is typical of nearly any man or woman who is anxious or depressed.

Physical Symptoms

The most frustrating part for me is not having a fixed timetable. When I had periods, I knew PMS only lasted a few days. But this process doesn't fit neatly into my calendar. How long will I have hot flashes? When will my periods stop? Is this going to last a year or two or ten? I think if I just knew, it would be easier to deal with, because right now this feels like a life sentence.

—Lana

HOT FLASHES

Hot flashes can vary in intensity, duration, and frequency. Hot flashes are caused by sudden changes in a woman's hormone levels, and symptoms include intense feelings of heat, sweating, rapid heartbeat, and flushing of the face. Keep a diary of your hot flashes. Hot flashes follow certain patterns. Certain things can trigger them, including hot weather, caffeine, and stress. When you keep track of your hot flashes for a week or two, you may discover the things that trigger them and then avoid or eliminate those triggers.

HYPNOSIS MIGHT HELP

The National Cancer Institute and NCCAM investigated the effects of hypnosis on hot flashes among women with a history of primary breast cancer and concluded that hypnosis appears to reduce perceived hot flashes in breast cancer survivors and may have additional benefits such as improved mood and sleep.

NONHORMONE MEDICATIONS

I did a lot of research and found that the antidepressant Effexor was successful in helping women with hot flashes. The study said this was especially of interest in women taking tamoxifen or other antiestrogens because of the hot flash side effects and no HT. So I began taking it, and it made a tremendous difference with mood stability and hot flashes. I felt normal again—well, normal mentally. I still have hot flashes, but they are much less frequent and much less severe. The antidepressant Paxil has also been studied for hot flashes, so women have a choice and may want to talk to their doctor and research the side effects of both drugs.

—Sally

In some cases, explains the North American Menopause Society, when women are unable or do not wish to take hormone therapy, nonhormonal prescription therapies which have been government-approved for other medical conditions have shown some efficacy in improving hot flashes. These drugs must be prescribed and adjusted carefully by your health care provider and include gabapentin, used to treat epilepsy and migraine; certain blood pressure medications; and low doses of some antidepressant medications (paroxetine, fluoxetine, and venlafaxine).

Ten Tips to Survive Hot Flashes

- Keep your core body temperature low.
- Turn down the thermostat by using a ceiling fan or air-conditioning.
- Dress in layers.
- Wear cotton, linen, or rayon clothes.
- Avoid wool, synthetic, and silk.
- Stick to open-necked shirts.
- Do relaxation exercises.
- Get a bigger bed if you and your partner are on different "heat planets."
- Take a cool shower before bed.
- Keep ice water at hand to drink and cool down from the inside.

PLANT-BASED TREATMENTS Some people successfully use herbs and other plants to treat hot flashes. Before you use them, talk to your doctor and ask about how it will interact with your other medications and treatment. Make sure you purchase only from a reputable source. Also, know that research studies have been mixed as to whether or not this form of treatment is effective. Some frequently used plant products include:

- **Black cohosh.** This used to be the gold standard in herbs for hormonal symptoms. Unfortunately, whether used alone or with other botanicals, it does not act like estrogen, as was once thought, and research done by the National Institute on Aging found that women taking black cohosh received no significant relief from their hot flashes and night sweats. In addition, women should discontinue the use of black cohosh and consult a health care practitioner if they have a liver disorder or develop symptoms of liver trouble, such as abdominal pain, dark urine, or jaundice.
- **Dong quai.** Only one randomized clinical study of dong quai has been done. The researchers did not find it to be useful in reducing hot flashes.
- **Soy extracts.** The scientific literature includes both positive and negative results on soy extracts for hot flashes. When taken for short periods of time, soy extracts appear to have few if any serious side effects. However, long-term use of soy extracts has been associated with thickening of the lining of the uterus.

SLEEP DISTURBANCES

Sleep is often disrupted by hot flashes, mood swings, anxiety, or other problems. You do have some control in how well you sleep, though. For example, drop the nap. Taking naps during the day can make it harder to fall asleep at night. Maintaining a regular bedtime schedule, including going to bed at the same time every night, helps sleep overall. Even what you eat can affect your sleep.

SLEEP-BOOSTING SNACKS Though a low-glycemic diet is ideal, carbohydrates can help you sleep. Try eating one of these about an hour before bedtime:

- Half of a whole wheat English muffin or raisin bagel drizzled with honey
- Two cups of air-popped popcorn
- A small slice of angel food cake topped with berries
- A frozen whole wheat waffle, toasted, with maple syrup
- Half a cup of pretzels
- Fresh strawberries dunked in a little fat-free chocolate syrup
- Half a cup of pasta topped with marinara sauce
- A four-ounce baked potato topped with salsa
- A handful of oyster crackers and a piece of fruit
- Canned mandarin oranges sprinkled with crystallized ginger

Spicy foods can raise your body temperature and disturb your beauty sleep. If you know that jalapeño nachos or hot mustard get you hot and bothered, give them up for dinner; just enjoy them at lunch.

LICORICE TEA

I usually have a cup of licorice tea in the evening about two hours before bed, and I don't have the sweats at night! I have noticed a general cooler body temperature. If I do get a bit hot, it isn't enough to cause those trickling sweat beads on my head/chest/back or enough to rudely interrupt my beauty sleep. So I'd say it really makes a difference for me. I just have to remember to drink it every night because on the nights I forget, I really regret it!

—Sharon

NIGHT SWEATS

Again I wake up, sweating, covers thrown off, and I have to pee. My night-clothes, sheets, and pillowcase contain as much moisture as the Amazon during a downpour. Anyone experiencing nighttime hot flashes knows damn well that simply removing the blankets is likely not enough to ease the discomfort. Getting naked doesn't even help. I don't think my sweats wake up my husband, but my thrashing around certainly does.

—Lisa

Sleep hyperhidrosis, otherwise known as "night sweats," happens to plenty of men and women because of a variety of medications or health conditions. It can also accompany hormone imbalances. Haralee Weintraub knows. A survivor of breast cancer, she started her own business making sleepwear for women going through night sweats after her own experiences.

"Most women wear the same old cotton T-shirt they've been wearing for several years. If you have night sweats, cotton is not your friend. Natural fibers like cotton retain moisture, and your clothes stick to you. You wake up cold and wet. For women with hot flashes who are suffering from night sweats, that is a major problem. You don't have to be miserable," explains Weintraub, the CEO of Haralee. Moisture-wicking fabric can be polyester, bamboo, or a poly/cotton blend. It is designed to pull moisture away from your skin to keep you dry. The fabric pushes moisture to its surface, where it is exposed to the night air and can evaporate quickly. The fabric is fast drying, easy to clean, and odor resistant. Pillowcases and bedsheets also come in wicking fabric.

When choosing nightwear, Wildbleu vice president Jay Delotte recommends putting on more fabric than less. Though it seems counterintuitive, he explains that the wicking fabric can pull moisture away only from skin that it is touching, so you'll want to wear sleepwear that hits traditional hot spots such as the back of your neck, your elbows, your cleavage, and behind your knees.

If none of the above tips helps, a sleep specialist might. The American Board of Sleep Medicine is the medical board that certifies sleep physicians and researchers as board-certified in sleep medicine. They maintain a searchable list of board-certified sleep specialists. See www.absm.org/diplomates/listing.htm.

INNOVATIVE PRODUCTS TO MAKE HOT FLASHES A LITTLE EASIER

MOISTURE-WICKING CLOTHING AND LINEN

WILDBLEU	www.wildbleu.com
HARALEE	www.haralee.com
DRYDREAMS	www.drydreamssleepwear.com
NITE SWEATZ	www.nitesweatz.com

OTHER PRODUCTS

The Chillow
www.chillowstore.com
The Chillow Sweet Relief Cooling Pillow Insert is a cooling and soothing device that cools you down without electricity.

The Bitty Breeze
www.thebittybreeze.com
Slim, foldaway fans in contemporary patterns that look much classier than waving a newspaper.

The Bed fan
www.bedfan.com
A small plug-in fan that attaches to your sheet to provide you with a constant, gentle flow of air.

Chili Pad
www.chilitechnology.com
This is the coolest mattress pad ever—literally. Think heated seats in luxury cars, but for your bed. But it can cool, too. Dual controls let you adjust the surface of your bed from 46 to 118 degrees. Soft silicon tubes move water throughout the mattress pad, and though it's pricey, a good night's sleep might well be worth it.

URINARY CONCERNS

The lower urinary tract is also impacted by low estrogen levels. It may seem as if every system in your body is affected by your hormones, which, while interesting, suddenly becomes a pain when your hormones are out of whack. Even peeing may become affected by what's happening with the rest of your body.

Urinary stress incontinence is the involuntary loss of bladder control. It usually occurs as a result of weakened muscles in the pelvic area due to age, childbirth, or, you got it, a lack of estrogen. Because those muscles have estrogen receptors, they lose their tone as estrogen receptors decline. The urethra, which passes urine out of the bladder, needs estrogen. With a decreased estrogen supply, the mucous lining of the urethra becomes thin, which causes the surrounding muscles to weaken.

You may not notice it at all until something happens that puts stress on your bladder, such as coughing, sneezing, laughing, or jogging. Those movements tug at the opening of the urethra, and if the muscles aren't strong enough, they can't resist the pull. The result? Loss of bladder control and the release of a small amount of urine. No, you do not need to go out and buy adult diapers; there are things you can do to help avoid an embarrassing accident.

Recent research has found that losing weight resulted in women's weekly urinary incontinence episodes being cut in half. "Losing weight, as part of a long-term strategy for healthy living including regular physical activity and eating a variety of food groups in moderation, can lead to significant results in reducing the severity of urinary leakage," says the Jean Hailes Foundation for Women's Health continence physiotherapist Janetta Webb. "This adds to the body of evidence that suggests making small changes toward a healthier lifestyle can have major benefits in overall quality of life."

There are other causes of urinary incontinence, so when you visit your health care provider, mention what's going on so other possibilities can be ruled out. Constipation, urinary tract infections, and medications such as sedatives, water pills (diuretics), muscle relaxants, and antidepressants can sometimes interfere with your ability to control your bladder function.

Low estrogen levels also affect the lining of the bladder. This can cause urinary frequency and even pain before and after urinating. It frequently makes women think they have a bladder infection even though no bacteria are present.

STRENGTHENING YOUR MUSCLES Do you know where your pubococcygeus (PC) muscles are? Or even what they are? In case you're wondering, they originate from your pubic bone, go under your genitals, and attach to your tailbone. Frankly, when it comes to physical fitness, most of us have never given this muscly matrix much thought. But we should. The PC muscles, like all muscles, begin to atrophy and wreak havoc of the kind that may eventually require the use of adult diapers. Seriously. And who needs incontinence issues when there are so many other aging-related matters to contend with down the road? Plus, stronger PC muscles not only mean fewer accidents, they mean better sex.

Kegel exercises strengthen your PC muscles, which support your uterus, bladder, and bowel. If you do Kegel exercises regularly and keep your muscles toned, you may reduce your risk of developing incontinence and similar problems as you get older. Kegel exercises may also be helpful to women who have persistent problems reaching orgasm. They aren't magic, but they do help strengthen your pelvic floor, the muscles that control your bladder, bowel, and sexual organs.

How to Do Kegels The secret to making Kegels work for you is to incorporate them into your daily routine. Every time your brush your teeth, do Kegels. Every time you stop at a red light, do Kegels. Create your own routine—whether it's when you take your vitamins, dry your hair, or check your e-mail.

Try to stop the flow of urine while you're going to the bathroom. If you succeed, you've got the basic move. The feeling is one of "squeeze and lift," a closing and drawing up of the front and back passages. Insert a clean finger into your vagina before doing a Kegel. If you feel pressure around your finger, you're on the right track. Or try a Kegel during love-making and ask your partner if he can feel it. If you're doing it correctly, he'll be able to feel you "hug" his penis. As your muscles become stronger and you become more experienced with the exercises, this movement will be more pronounced.

Don't make a habit of starting and stopping your urine stream. Doing Kegel exercises with a full bladder or while emptying your bladder can actually weaken the muscles. It can also lead to incomplete emptying of the bladder, which increases your risk of a urinary tract infection. If you're having trouble finding the right muscles, don't be embarrassed to ask your doctor for help. He or she can provide feedback so that you can learn to isolate and exercise the correct muscles.

Perfect Your Technique Once you've identified your PC muscles, empty your bladder and get into a sitting or standing position. Then firmly tense your PC muscles. Try to do so at frequent intervals for five seconds at a time, four or five times in a row. Work up to keeping the muscles contracted for ten seconds at a time, relaxing for ten seconds between contractions. Also, try not to hold your breath. Just relax, breathe freely, and focus on tightening the muscles around your vagina and rectum.

Perform a set of ten Kegel exercises at least three times a day. The exercises will get easier the more often you do them. Do Kegels:

- Whenever you are at a red light
- During commercials
- While you brush your teeth
- While you listen to phone messages
- While you wait for the snooze alarm to go off again
- Just before bed
- During sex
- While waiting in line

- While checking your e-mail
- While doing relaxation exercises

Vary your technique. Try doing sets of mini-Kegels. Count quickly to ten or twenty, contracting and relaxing your pelvic floor muscles each time you say a number. Or slow down, gradually contracting and releasing your pelvic floor muscles once. As you contract, visualize an elevator traveling up four floors. At each floor, contract your muscles a little more until you reach maximum contraction at the fourth floor. Hold the contraction and then slowly release the tension as you visualize the elevator traveling back down. Repeat ten times.

WEIGHTS FOR MY WHAT? Weighted vaginal cones can be used to help strengthen the PC muscles. They come in a set of five reusable, tamponlike, sterile cones of identical size and shape but of increasing weight. The tapered end of the cone is inserted into the vagina, and you contract your PC muscles to try to hold it in so that it doesn't slip out of the vagina. As the muscles get stronger, you progress to a heavier cone. Several brands even come with video instructions.

These aren't cheap. You're going to spend between $60 and $100, and you aren't going to want to buy these puppies used. You don't need a prescription, and you can purchase them online from such retailers as www.vaginalweights.net and www.shopinprivate.com. Here are some tips:

- Start with the cone that you can hold for one minute.
- Do the exercise twice a day.
- Gradually increase the length of time that you can hold the cone in place, until you can hold it for fifteen minutes.
- You can then increase the weight or use the next heaviest cone.
- Continue until you can use the heaviest cone in the set for fifteen minutes, twice a day.

We know that weights for your vagina may seem a little . . . unusual, but studies show that they work. Like any exercise, the more you do these, the better the results. They take a real commitment in time and effort, though.

Do not use vaginal cones or weights if:

- You are pregnant and have a history of miscarriage or have been advised to avoid sex
- Your vulva or vagina is inflamed or infected
- You have a moderate or severe vaginal prolapse (where the front wall of your vagina and part of your bladder drop down into the entrance of your vagina)
- You are menstruating
- You've had sexual intercourse within the last two hours
- You've had pelvic surgery in the last three months

SKIN CARE

I have constantly dry skin. I pay out the wazoo for really good skin care with extra moisturizing, plus foundation with moisturizer. My only luxury is skin care.

—Lorin

Why can't low estrogen levels do anything fantastic, such as make your skin perfectly smooth and glorious? Low estrogen and pro-gesterone levels create thinner, looser, and less elastic skin, reduced collagen production, cessation of oil gland function, and dry skin. Caring for your skin will require some extra effort to maintain that dewy, youthful look you love.

Dry Skin Care Tips
- **Add a teaspoon of oil** to your salads, salad dressings, and cooking in the form of olive oil, safflower oil, coconut oil, or flaxseed oil, which are especially high in omega-3 fatty acids and excellent for the hair, nails, and skin.
- **Drink up.** Drink eight to ten glasses of water a day, more if you perform intense exercise. Water will cleanse your body and skin of the bad toxins and chemicals that dry it out.
- **Have some green tea.** Scientific studies show that green tea extract is extremely high in antioxidants. These protect the body

from free radicals, natural particles in the body that accelerate the aging process.

- **Sleep well.** Aim for at least eight hours of sleep per night.
- **Ditch unnecessary chemicals.** Switch to a natural cleanser that is free of chemicals that will dry out your skin.

Anything that further dries your skin, such as overuse of soaps, antiperspirants, perfumes, or hot baths, will make the problem worse. Dehydration, sun exposure, smoking, and stress may also cause dry skin. Protection against the UVA and UVB rays of the sun is a must to prevent skin damage.

Though you may not have a lot of choices about your medications, you can choose what skin care products you put on your body. Mary Cuneo, the co-owner of Grateful Body skin care products, says, "Reclaiming our relationship with our bodies is so important. Choosing handcrafted products made with pure botanical oils and slow-tinctured herbal blends literally feeds your skin and offers enough nourishment that your skin can balance and heal itself. Our bodies respond when we do something good for them." Several companies provide natural skin care products especially designed for very dry skin, including:

Grateful Body, www.gratefulbody.com
Skin Organics, www.skinorganicsaw.com
Emerita, www.emerita.com

Contrary to rumor, applying soy extract, black cohosh, wild yam, or evening primrose oil to your skin isn't going to replace what your body needs for better skin. They aren't dangerous—a dab of black cohosh in your moisturizer won't hurt you—but their benefits are most likely not different from those of other anti-inflammatory and antioxidant cosmetic ingredients.

NAIL CARE

Some women notice that as their estrogen levels drop, their fingernails become drier and more brittle. Dr. Paul Kechijian, an associate clinical professor of dermatology and chief of the nail section at New York University Medical Center in New York City, offers these tips for healthier nails:

- Apply moisturizer to your hands every time you wash them—or any other time they've been in water.
- Keep your fingernails on the short side to prevent damage and breakage.
- Wear gloves if it is cold enough to wear a jacket.
- Limit your use of nail polish remover to once a week.

Milagro nail care products are formulated to make stronger fingernails. The same people who make shampoo for dry and damaged hair have created nail care products that you may find useful; plus they dry in just ten seconds!

HAIR CHANGES

I can deal with the symptoms. I can. None of these are a big deal; I just try to tell myself that I am becoming higher maintenance as I age. I was never one to spend a ton on makeup or skin creams, but I won't leave the house without a tweezer now. Those chin hairs sprout in minutes—you think I'm kidding, but I'm not. I am also an expert on hair care products now. It doesn't feel as full as it used to, but the biggest change I see is that it isn't as shiny. That's okay, though, because the salon sells stuff for that, too. I can either focus on being miserable or I can decide I am worth the extra time and attention I now require to look beautiful.

—Toni

Seriously, this too? Some women (about a third of those who experience decreased estrogen levels) will experience changes in their hair. (This can include hair loss as well as excessive hair growth.) The hair on your head may seem less glossy, and it may even thin out some. But you usually won't go bald unless you have other serious health problems going on, too. To restore some of the sheen, try these tips:

- Stop the perms and bleaching.
- Use very gentle shampoos.
- Apply a weekly deep conditioner.

- Pat your hair dry.
- If you have to blow-dry, use a thermal conditioner.
- Use sunscreen made for hair.

Spend some time on message boards, and you'll find that a few names pop up time and time again. Nisim International makes a popular shampoo, and some women swear by it for keeping hair longer and stronger. My favorite part? The money-back guarantee. Go to www .nisim.com.

On the other hand, the wiry, thick hair that grows in your pubic area and your armpits may get darker and thicker and show up in some unusual places, such as your chin or abdomen. Bleaching, waxing, and electrolysis or laser therapy can all do wonders for those.

DRY EYES

I have really sensitive eyes now. I am more sensitive to light than I used to be. There's definitely the sense that any extra moisture has just drained out of my body.

—Bonnie

Estrogen levels can also affect your eyes and give you dry eyes, a condition in which the moisture normally covering the eye is lacking in quality, quantity, or both. Dr. Robert Latkany of Physician Eyecare of New York is the author of the book *The Dry Eye Remedy* and suggests these tips to help reduce the symptoms of dry eyes.

- Wear sunglasses, eyeglasses, or a hat when you are outside.
- Do not leave your ceiling fan on at night.
- Remember to blink when you are reading, working on the computer, or doing any task that requires concentration.
- Prescription medication is available, but it can take up to a month to feel any changes.
- Artificial tears are safe to use three to four times a day and are preferred by patients who do not want to take prescription medicine.

It is possible to have ovarian insufficiency and feel beautiful and calm once again. You may need to spend some extra time and money to look your best, but you aren't doomed to looking as though you're old enough to go through menopause when you're not. If we can cultivate increased self-acceptance and take good care of ourselves, the way we feel about ourselves will naturally improve.

PART FOUR

Living Well

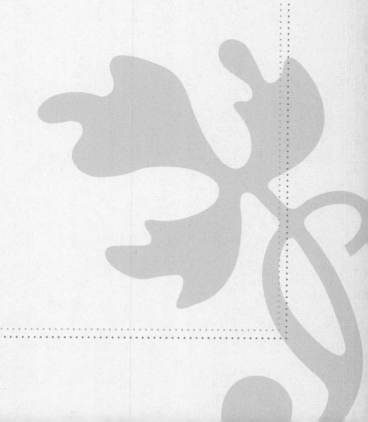

12

Accept Your Emotions

The best advice anyone gave me: don't make any rush decisions.
Upon learning your diagnosis, you will probably go through a series
of emotions, including denial, devastation, regret, anger, and/or
depression. It takes time before your body and mind have time to
adjust to your situation. Wait until then before you make any major
decisions about what you want to do with your life, particularly
concerning children.

Upon diagnosis, I felt I had to immediately have a child and do it
in any way I could—adoption or donor egg or whatever, I didn't
care. That heightened emotional state is not a good frame of mind
to be in when making a real decision. Be sure you have carefully
thought out all your options and given yourself time to heal and
accept your diagnosis before embarking on other changes that such
a decision as adding a child to your life will bring.

—Tina

EVERY ASPECT OF A woman's life is impacted by a diagnosis of ovarian insufficiency. For many young women, the realization that their fertility has been affected is quite upsetting, says Karin A. Clark, the director of the Center for Conceiving Health. "You have to accept that it is likely dreams you have held forever about your life will not happen the way you might have envisioned. You may well doubt your femininity and womanhood and watch your trust in your own body dissolve, at least for a while. Long-held beliefs and views of the world and reality will be called into question.

"And faith? Whatever that meant before, there is no way it won't be called into question. In other words, once you receive this news, the descent into an existential crisis of monumental proportions is likely inevitable. Giving yourself permission to embrace, despite the irony of that word, this crisis and move all the way into and through it is the only possible way to truly heal. Anything less is unlikely to offer you a full and joyful life on the other side."

Emotional well-being during early menopause can be influenced by many factors, including:

- Personality
- Life experiences—trauma and illness, for example
- Individual thinking and behavior patterns
- Earlier mood problems, such as depression and anxiety
- Lifestyle: health, stress, activity, substance use
- Self-esteem; your roles and sense of purpose in life
- Body image
- Relationships; family and support networks
- Faith—or belief in a higher purpose in life

Dealing with a Diagnosis

"The term 'premature ovarian failure' has always struck me the wrong way—especially because it has the word 'failure' in it," says Dr. Marcelle Pick. "I know receiving a diagnosis of premature ovarian failure is heartbreaking. I also know that it takes time to heal and understand what your life will look like afterwards. Give yourself time. But also understand that you haven't failed. In the end, your body deserves the best health you can give it. Do this by learning more, taking care to prevent the health risks associated with ovarian insufficiency and finding true happiness. Release yourself from what you thought would happen and create a new life picture, one that satisfies your goals and desires."

"Many women feel a sense of urgency to act right away when they get their diagnosis," National Institutes of Health (NIH) researcher Dr. Lawrence Nelson says. But, based on his years of experience, he suggests a slower, more deliberate plan to his patients for dealing with infertility related to POI. Dr. Nelson has been caring for women who have POI for decades. As the head of the NIH's Integrative Reproductive Medicine

Unit, he is working to understand POI and to help women and families affected by it.

First, he recommends that women allow themselves time to feel and deal with the emotions that may accompany a diagnosis of POI. He explains that becoming emotionally healthy, no matter how long it takes, is the best way to prepare for the tough decisions that may be down the road. Karin A. Clark agrees. "Grappling with a diagnosis as devastating as POI is likely to be nearly impossible to digest for a period of time. Giving yourself the time you need—likely months for the initial shock and then grief to wash through you—is imperative to be able to truly move on in your life without harboring a sea of bitterness."

Next, Dr. Nelson suggests that women focus on their relationships with their spouses, partners, and families. Resources for strengthening those relationships can be found in later chapters. In addition, the help of a professional listener is very important in building strong, close relationships after a POI diagnosis.

You Aren't Crazy

> *My mom joked once with my dad that if she didn't know different she would have said I was going through the menopause at the time she was going through the same. However, Mom also shared the same joke with my specialist, who, rather than trying to find out what on earth was going on with me, referred me to a psychiatrist, as I was obviously seeking attention and mimicking my mother's symptoms. I really thought I was going mad and that I was imagining these symptoms. By this point I was fourteen and heading into my final two years at school. All I wanted was to feel like a normal teenager talking about boys and enjoying music rather than discussing hot flushes with my mom.*
>
> —Christine

Loss and Grief

When ovarian insufficiency or menopause do not come at the expected age and stage of life, they may impact well-being more significantly. Associated illnesses, such as cancer and chemotherapy or surgery to remove ovaries, may also alter the course of one's life. Grief and loss can be more pronounced. Not only is there the loss of control, ability to plan, and self-image, but often there is no one with whom to share grief.

Girlfriends may not understand because they are not yet experiencing menopause, and for some, their mothers haven't reached menopause either. In fact, it may take some time to diagnose an early menopause. Not knowing what is wrong, having no control over symptoms, and not knowing what the future holds can be truly frightening. Some women with early menopause talk of "loss of womanhood" and "loss of dreams" in their twenties and thirties with fifty to sixty years left of their life to live.

> *When I was told I had gone through menopause at twenty-two years of age, I couldn't even talk to my mother about it because she hadn't even gone through menopause herself. It was important to find someone who understood my situation.*
>
> —Kate

It is really important to identify and work through your feelings. To do this, it is important to find a way to say how you're feeling—are you frustrated, angry, sad? Talking, writing in a journal or diary, drawing, and physical activities such as walking and yoga are all good ways of getting feelings and thoughts out.

Self-esteem

Self-esteem is what we believe about ourselves, how we value and respect ourselves. Self-esteem can be influenced by the roles we have in life, our relationships, and our experiences. Ultimately, self-esteem comes down to whether we acknowledge our successes and put our "failures" into perspective. If we always focus on what we can't do, we are likely to feel bad about ourselves. This is important when it comes to ovarian insufficiency or early menopause. If you feel that you are a failure or not successful at anything and focus only on this, your self-esteem will be low.

Challenge these thoughts and feelings and focus on things that you can do—and do well. You may be a fantastic friend, or you may be really creative or good in the garden or at cooking. Everyone has something she is good at, and you need to acknowledge these things. If you truly can't think of something, then now is the time to dream and add new activities and roles. Low self-esteem is a big contributor to feelings of anxiety and depression, so it can be really helpful to work through this with a mental health professional.

The Blues

It's easy to feel blue when your body isn't working right. Having a physical illness can sometimes cause you to feel down. But if the sadness is severe or long-lasting, you may be experiencing clinical depression along with your medical condition. This is called "co-occurring" depression. Clinical depression is a serious but treatable illness. Depression is more likely to occur along with certain other medical illnesses and conditions, such as cancer, heart disease, and—you got it—hormone disorders! The good news is that people who are treated for co-occurring depression usually experience improvement in their overall medical condition and a better quality of life. Plus, they find they are more willing to follow their medical care guidelines.

Check out these depression-screening guidelines to and see if your blues warrant a call to your health care provider.

DEPRESSION SCREENING

If you have been experiencing five or more of the below symptoms for more than two weeks, if suicide is a serious concern, or if the symptoms are severe enough to interfere with a daily routine, see your doctor or qualified mental health professional.

- Persistent sad, anxious, or "empty" mood
- Sleeping too much or too little; middle-of-night or early-morning waking
- Reduced appetite and weight loss or increased appetite and weight gain
- Loss of pleasure and interest in activities once enjoyed, including sex
- Irritability, restlessness
- Persistent physical symptoms that do not respond to treatment (such as chronic pain or digestive disorders)
- Difficulty concentrating, remembering, or making decisions
- Fatigue or loss of energy
- Feeling guilty, hopeless, or worthless
- Thoughts of death or suicide

Source: National Mental Health Association.

Get Help

> *I did not want to be rejected by a potential mate and I did not want to face not being able to give a future husband a family, so I established a career focus. I dated very little and worked hard on pursuing my master's degree and achieving success in my chosen profession. I am now forty and have had many happy experiences; I don't regret my decision. However, if I were doing it again I might have sought some counseling in my twenties to give me strategies for experiencing a more complete social life.*
>
> —Serena

Obviously, while there may be some cultural pressures and expectations, there is no need to have a partner to feel complete. However, most people prefer to be in a loving, functional relationship when given the opportunity. Fear that you may be rejected because of the potential difficulty of having children or a lack of sexual feelings may stop you from pursuing an intimate relationship. Getting counseling may be the right step for you to help you make life decisions after you have your diagnosis.

Self Care

Taking care of yourself doesn't necessarily happen easily. We all have competing demands for our time, energy, and attention. However, once we realize that our physical and emotional selves are connected, we may be more willing to take care of our emotional, social, and spiritual needs. Need some ideas? Start with these:

- Keep a journal.
- Take a walk (sunshine and vitamin D are good for you!).
- Spend some time with a dog or cat.
- Get a massage.
- Pick up an old hobby, or start a new one.
- Call a friend.
- Sing (in the car, in the shower—just be loud!).
- Find a community (church, volunteer organization, social group, etc.).
- Make the world look better by planting something.
- Watch a movie or read a book designed to make you laugh.

Find Faith

Though it may not feel like it at this moment, there is more to life than this diagnosis. It can feel overwhelming at times, so it is important to continue to build healthy relationships, develop outside interests, and take excellent care of yourself—physically, emotionally, and spiritually.

13

Build Relationships

Many people suspect my condition, but because premature menopause is a closed issue, they don't like to ask. And I don't rush in and confide in others. If my work colleagues knew I was menopausal and unable to have children, then they would feel uncomfortable, especially talking about their children. My husband has been a great support and accompanied me on my journey. In fact, if it had not been for him, I know I would have crumbled a long time ago.

—Sharyn

IT SEEMS AS THOUGH your hormones affect everything from your bladder to sex life, even your sleep and dental health. Did we mention your bones and heart health? It hardly seems fair that your ovary dysfunction can affect your relationships, too. This time, the cause isn't necessarily biological. Your relationships with your significant other, friends, even work colleagues may be affected at times by what you are experiencing physically.

Dating Relationships

It made relationships difficult. When do you tell a boyfriend that you can't have children, when you first go out with him? That will terrify him, but if you leave it too late you run the risk of it seeming as if you've kept something hidden—and who talks about having children at eighteen?

—Fay

The stresses and symptoms that can accompany ovarian insufficiency can have a significant impact on how a woman views herself. Ultimately, this can have an impact on relationships with a partner, if you have one. Some women who go through ovarian insufficiency or early menopause are not yet in a committed relationship, and this can provide another challenge. How do you tell a new partner that you have gone through "menopause" (because who else would know what ovarian insufficiency is?) at twenty years of age and you might not be able to have children? As Toni asks, "How can I tell a future partner that I have already gone through menopause? I don't even know what to say when I have a hot flash. Somehow, fanning myself with sweat dripping down my face and laughing it off as a 'power surge' doesn't feel right."

What exactly does it look like to tell someone you're dating that your reproductive health isn't actually up to snuff? When do you tell? Does it look like this?

"I don't usually answer personal ads, either."

"It's good to meet you."

"So, where are you from?"

"What do you do?"

"That sounds interesting. By the way, I have this condition where my ovaries don't work anymore and I'm not that interested in sex and sometimes I have hot flashes and I'll probably need professional help to get pregnant. Did I mention some pretty wild mood swings when I start switching my medication around?"

"Where did you go?"

"Hello?"

So maybe you don't tell someone on the first date. Maybe not even on the second or third. Certainly, there is some fear that if you disclose your health status too early in the process of forming a relationship, the other person will be scared away. On the other hand, others may see it as a test: "Here I am, take me or leave me." Deciding how soon to tell depends on your comfort level. There is no one perfect answer: "You must submit a medical report by the fourth date or before you go to second base."

There will come a point in any relationship that is moving toward permanent life partnership where you will need to inform your partner of what you're facing, if only because he or she will be facing those difficulties too, and to keep him or her in the dark at that point would be problematic. As hard as it is, do not expect the perfect response immediately. You have had some time to deal with your diagnosis, and your initial reaction may not have been terrifically heroic or brave. Let your partner know it may be difficult information to process, ask if he or she has any questions, and suggest you talk about it again the next time you get together after he or she has had time to process the information.

HOW PARTNERS CAN OFFER SUPPORT

He constantly reassured me that I was not old in either looks or behavior; that was my most difficult hurdle. He was always there for me when I wanted to talk, but he never pushed me to talk to him about it.

—Lani

Knowing what to say or do when a loved one is facing a health challenge is difficult. There are no magic words guaranteed to make life easier, no script or playbook to tell you what to say or do next. Some of these phrases are good places to start:

"I don't know what to say."
"I'm sorry you are hurting/scared."
"What do you need me from right now?"
"I can tell you are really upset."

Friends and Family

I can tell you that my family and friend relationships are a little bit different. Just a few people in my family know I have this, so sometimes they wonder why I don't come out and play with their six-year-old or want to hold the newborn. Other times, even my immediate family forgets that I have a bit of a hard time being around babies and toddlers, and they can be a bit insensitive at times.

—Susan

It may come as a surprise, but people with whom you are close and have had good relationships with for years may completely botch up being supportive. They may say the wrong things:

- "You can always adopt."
- "Look on the bright side: you're so lucky not to have to worry about periods anymore."

- Or the old favorite, "Kids are a hassle—you can always have one of mine." I always wanted to say, "Really? That's great. Can I pick which one? I'll be by tomorrow morning to pick her up; what time works for you?"

The last thing you need during this time is other people's well-meaning input. Karin A. Clark warns, "Beware of any sentence beginning with 'At least . . . ' 'At least now you have an answer and you can let go.' Another real favorite is 'At least it isn't life-threatening.' While I have never done it, I have always wished I could say, 'Really? I wouldn't be so sure. If you said that to me when I was faced with an issue that painful, I can imagine feeling slightly homicidal.'"

Don't fall into the trap of believing you should listen or be polite and understanding about some well-wisher's intention. There are two ways to consider handling this. One is to put your hand up before he or she gets any farther into the sentence and say gently, "Please, I am not looking for advice. I am working through this in my own way. Thanks for caring, though." If you would rather have your fingernails pulled out than be that "confrontational" or assertive, the second option is to have a thought planted in your head to refer to when someone opens their mouth with advice, something like "Their opinion has nothing to do with my reality or what is best for me." Because that's the truth.

Identify Your Needs

Trust yourself. You know how you feel both physically and emotionally. Trust the people who are close to you and love you. Tell them how you feel if you think it might help you to deal with this. If your parents try to make you feel guilty that you can't give them grandchildren, remind them that this was not your choice. . . . The people who love you really do love you! They care, but the things that cause them pain about your POF are different than the things that cause you pain. Help them to understand, because, in my experience, once they understand, they are a wonderful, stable, strong place to rest and be just yourself.

—Winnie

Because ovarian dysfunction is unusual enough that it isn't mainstream, plenty of people will offer advice that has absolutely nothing to do with your particular situation, sometimes even assuring you that doctors are idiots, lab tests can be wrong, and everything will be just fine. All those things may well be true, but that doesn't negate the fact that your experience is painful now and what you need is understanding.

> *I finally had to tell my best friend that all of the stories of miracle babies weren't helping me right now. Right now I'm just really sad about my diagnosis and I need to just cry and complain for a little while. She was okay with that—she thought I wanted to hear all happy, encouraging news to cheer me up. Soon, I hope, but I'm not quite there yet. Now she just brings Kleenex and a pint of ice cream. Perfect.*
>
> —Ellen

Some friends or family may withdraw because they don't know how to respond and assume that saying nothing is better than saying the wrong thing. Unfortunately, you may end up feeling isolated and alone, as if no one cares. Not everyone will be able to give you what you need. Other people will care and want to be helpful, but you may have to let them know what you need.

LISTEN TO OTHERS' NEEDS

Wild mood swings, anxiety about treatment options, fears about the future—sometimes our concerns and fears spill over into our other relationships. Though it is natural to want to hunker down when dealing with what feels like a crisis, don't ignore the people in your life who are reaching out to you. Acknowledge that you might be difficult to be with at times, show your appreciation for loving-kindnesses, and accept support from a number of different sources so you don't completely drain one person.

Long-term Relationship Issues

> *For me, the diagnosis of POI, which came almost two years after my husband and I split up, was a relief. It was real. It was not in my mind. I was not a hypochondriac. Plus, now I could see how POI affected our relationship. My emotions, my lack of sex drive, even trying to get pregnant all took their toll. I wonder if an earlier diagnosis would have saved our marriage?*
>
> —Grace

It might be that, as a couple, you need to define or redefine your goals, expectations, dreams, and plans. Partners also need to be aware of what is happening, both physically and psychologically. Couples dealing with fertility issues, the possibility of having or not having a family, plans, and expectations need to be able to talk openly. Low libido and mood swings can affect even the healthiest relationship. Just as your diagnosis affects you, it affects the people you are in a relationship with. Whether the issue is a change in your level of physical intimacy or adjusting to the new reality, many couples find it beneficial to seek an outside source of professional help. It may also be helpful for partners to read this book so they can better understand what you are going through.

> *I realized I was picking fights with Mike, just trying to get him to leave me. I still thought he deserved a wife who didn't have the reproductive plumbing of a ninety-year-old. I guess I thought if he wouldn't leave me of his own accord, then I would push him until he had no other choice. I always say Mike's either a crazy man or he really loves me, because he never left. He took the crazy ride with me. I decided that I had to stop picking at him. I deserved a good husband, and he deserved a nonpsycho wife. Going into therapy helped us keep it together.*
>
> —Kayla

HOW TO FIND A RELATIONSHIP THERAPIST

The National Registry of Marriage Friendly Therapists was developed to help marriages by linking couples with the most highly qualified therapists in the country. Marriage friendly therapists are unrelated to any religious or political organization, so you can find marriage counseling across the spectrum from secular to religious. The marriage counselors also practice many models of counseling, representing a wide range of marriage therapy styles. See www.marriagefriendly therapists.com.

14

Reclaim Your Sexuality

*A recent study found that 30 percent of women said that sex was
actually better after menopause. I think that may be due to the
memory loss. I'm not saying we forget how good it used to be but that
we forget where we live and end up having sex with strangers.*

—Leigh Anne Jasheway-Bryant, author of
Not Guilty by Reason of Menopause

IF ONLY IT WERE as simple as that. For many women, sexuality during
and after ovarian dysfunction becomes more complicated. Even if you
find great sex, you still might have hot flashes, a lower libido, and vaginal lubrication issues. But just because you may have a few new hurdles
in the bedroom doesn't mean you need to give up physical intimacy.
You might need to be a little more creative and learn a few new tricks.
Research shows that orgasms are good for overall well-being—both
physically and mentally. An integral part of a healthy life is a healthy sex
life. Now, let's help you get there!

*I have a good sex life. I work at it, and it takes more effort than for most women,
but I enjoy it! Despite a loving and wonderful husband, my sex drive was lower
than zero. None. At first it was no big deal, but I started approaching my one-
year mark. My feelings for him were still the same, but I had no interest in sex,
kissing, etc. I just didn't care if I ever had sex again, and I decided I was not
willing to live the rest of my life like that. I decided to do some research, and
now I drive two hours to a different doctor, but it's getting better.*

—Cindy

What's a Girl to Do?

Hormone levels decrease when ovaries become insufficient, regardless of when it happens. Dwindling hormones affect many areas of your life, and sex is one of them. Going through ovarian insufficiency at an early age doesn't have to mean the end of your sex life, but you will probably have to make some adjustments.

The younger you are when you begin experiencing symptoms, the sooner you may start to experience some problems. The symptoms vary, but if you have ovarian dysfunction, you may notice decreased desire, vaginal dryness that causes painful intercourse, and difficulty having an orgasm. While you may have to make some changes in expectations, you don't have to give up having a satisfying intimate physical relationship. Your sexuality is still largely within your control.

Find Your Sexual Self

Entering menopause so early has given me serious body issues about feeling nonfeminine. I mean, on one hand, it's just my ovaries, not me. But there are times when I sort of feel asexual, as if I wasn't really one gender or the other. If I don't have periods, don't make my own hormones, and am not that interested in sex right now, what is it that makes me a woman?

—Wendy

What does it mean to feel feminine? Is it being able to get pregnant? Is it feeling beautiful or at least attractive? Or does it have more to do with feeling the desire to be sexually intimate?

Women who experience ovarian insufficiency or early menopause, particularly when it is surgically induced, can experience a significant change in their view of their bodies. The sudden drop in hormones with surgery may make a woman feel that her body is totally out of control. This can also bring symptoms that are frustrating, annoying, confusing, and distressing. It is not surprising that women talk of not being able to trust their body and seeing their body in a more negative way. Some don't feel as attractive or desirable.

I know it's tough—any and all of us who've dealt with this whole POI/POF thing has grappled with the "Am I still sexy? Am I still a woman? Am I still what

I thought I was?" stuff. And from one who's been there and come out the other end (I married after being diagnosed with POF), all I want to share with you is that you're so much more than ovaries or ability to procreate or whatever. I know, I know . . . it's easy for me to say since I've gotten past it—but it's true.

—Lisa

A young body is not supposed to behave like this, and women often say, "I am a young woman in an older woman's body." Dry skin, a dry vagina, and increased risk of osteoporosis are significant changes to experience in your twenties and thirties. It is important that all these aspects be acknowledged, discussed, and understood in some way if they are having an impact on you.

Your body will go through some subtle and not-so-subtle changes with ovarian insufficiency. Your weight may fluctuate, your skin may change, and your sexual responsiveness may even change. But the biggest difference may be in your head. A lot of the symptoms can be treated with medical interventions, complementary medicine, or lifestyle changes. But how you feel about yourself and what it means to be a woman is up to you, and to some extent, your partner.

Tina, a young woman who battled breast cancer, put it this way: "Cancer and the treatment threaten every facet of your femininity. Chemo makes you lose your hair. Chemo may make me lose my *fingernails*. Until now my fingernails were the most perfect part of my body. The mastectomy takes your breasts. Chemo causes premature menopause. Menopause at thirty-three! I am not missing my periods, but I find it crazy that the magazines I am drawn to at the gyn's office are menopause magazines with articles on dealing with hot flashes. My top concern at thirty-three should be birth control, not menopause. I shouldn't be going through menopause at the same time as my mom.

"So, since my feminine side is being attacked, I am becoming more feminine. I have bought quite a bit of makeup lately. (I'm still not wearing it, but now I have it if my eyebrows totally fall out.) I wear skirts often. I have lots of lovely hats. I have a beautiful wig. I don't have the option of just copping out and wearing a ponytail every day; I have to consider how to dress my head. I even find I match my headwear to the clothes I am wearing. I find myself reading blogs and postings of other courageous, beautiful women for at least an hour every day. I spent the first half of my life wanting to surround myself with boys and all things masculine. Now I find myself longing for the feminine and needing to connect with all things female."

Remember, being a woman is not defined by your hormone levels or which body parts are working. How you decide to perceive your changing body will have dramatic effects on your outlook. This is where you must take responsibility for getting the support you need. Discuss what you need with your partner. Find women going through similar struggles. Do not allow yourself to wallow in negative thinking (the occasional pity party is allowed—you just can't take up residence there).

Where's My Libido?

I never thought I would say this, but I have totally lost interest in sex. I don't even think about it. But even when I do, it seems like too much trouble. I feel sterile, old, dried up, and sexless at too early an age. I am only thirty-eight, and if I don't have sex this month, that's fine with me.

—Lisa

I'M JUST TOO SAD TO THINK ABOUT SEX

Remember: not only is depression a major cause of decreased libido and sexual satisfaction, but decreased libido and decreased sexual satisfaction are early symptoms of depression. Ovarian insufficiency may be accompanied by feelings of loss of identity and a crisis of femininity; it may also bring with it a myriad of other emotional issues. A host of changing emotions may lead you to feel withdrawn and isolated from your friends.

It's one thing not to want sex after you have had a pretty hot sex life for thirty-five years, but what if you're just starting to get your sexual groove on?

One of the main differences between undergoing ovarian insufficiency early is how you experience your sex life with your partner. If you're well into your fifties or sixties, for example, a decreased libido may not be much of a problem, because your partner is often around the same age and also may have decreased desire. In fact, by age sixty-five about 20 percent of men have erectile dysfunction one out of every four times they have sex. This may happen in men with heart disease, high blood pressure, or diabetes, because of either the disease or the medicines used to treat it. When systems fail, operators are less likely to want to boot up as often. But if you're thirty and trying to maintain an active sex life, it can be a different story. You and your partner may have very different expectations than an older couple does about what a "normal" sex life should be. What can you do if your libido tanks?

MEDICATIONS MATTER

Keep in mind that some medications affect libido, so talk to your physician about possible side effects of any and all medications you are already taking or are considering. Some medications, such as those for depression/anxiety or high blood pressure, can also affect your sex drive. There may be alternatives you can switch to if necessary. Chronic conditions such as diabetes, sleep apnea, and pituitary problems can also play a role.

Again, see your physician to create a treatment plan that addresses all areas of your health, including sexual. If you're not comfortable talking to your physician about sex, write down a list of questions. Or if the problem is the doctor and not you, you might want to find a less uptight physician or one who is more knowledgeable.

CHANGING YOUR LIFESTYLE
TO BOOST YOUR SEX DRIVE

While we all wish there was a magic pill that would boost our sex drive, it just doesn't exist. A woman's lack of sexual interest is often tied to her relationship with her partner, says Sandra Leiblum, the director for sexual and marital health at the Robert Wood Johnson Medical School. "The important sex organ [for women] is between the ears. Men need a place for having sex; women need a purpose." Low libido at any stage of a woman's life can be triggered by family concerns, illness or death, financial or job worries, child care responsibilities, managing a career and children, previous or current physical and emotional abuse, fatigue, and depression. We're not wired to be passive victims of hormonal dysfunction.

"You can have a woman with low hormone levels change partners and suddenly her libido is just fine, or you can have a woman with great hormone levels who is in a lousy relationship, or who is suffering from depression, and her desire is basically blotto," says Dr. Glenn D. Braunstein, an endocrinologist and chairman of the Department of Medicine at Cedars Sinai Medical Center in Los Angeles.

Besides hormones, what else can adversely impact your sex life? Drinking alcohol, smoking cigarettes, and using marijuana or other illegal drugs can all dampen your enthusiasm, so if you've been looking for a reason to quit, increased libido is a good one. Or it may be you're not getting enough sleep. "Poor sleep can reduce energy for everything, including sex," according to Dr. Susan D. Reed, associate professor of obstetrics and gynecology and epidemiology at the University of Washington.

Vaginal Dryness and Painful Intercourse

I've had issues with vaginal dryness, a really bad episode when changing HT a while back, and sex was so painful it was out of the question. He was very nervous to have sex again even when I was feeling better because of the pain I had been in, and that caused some challenges but also some very open dialogue on lovemaking and intimacy and created a closer emotional connection.

—Meg

The lining of the vagina is pink, plump, and juicy when it is full of estrogen. But when the estrogen level starts to fall, the lining grows thinner and makes sex less enjoyable. Maintaining healthy vaginal tissue makes a big difference in your ability to respond to and have orgasms. Dryness and pain often occur due to low estrogen levels in the tissues of the vagina.

Why? Some women describe sex as "a sandpaper-like feeling when he enters me," or they feel stinging on entry of the penis. Some women think they were well lubricated during sex because there is still a watery moistness but feel a stinging when they urinate afterward. That means there has been a tear. Microscopic tears build up and then invite bacteria and infection in. It's a vicious cycle.

The vaginal tissue stops lubricating the way it did before menopause. Dr. Monica Peacocke, a scientist and vaginal specialist in New York, describes the difference between "good lubrication" and "bad lubrication." The good kind is the thick, slippery mucus that flows during sexual arousal in women who still have normal estrogen levels or are using hormone replacement. "Bad lubrication" is thin and watery due to the decreased estrogen after menopause, and while it may feel like normal moistness, it does not smooth the channel for the penis.

Without estrogen, the vagina is less lubricated and the vaginal lining is thinner. Lower estrogen levels also decrease the blood supply to the vagina and the surrounding nerves, making the vagina drier. These symptoms may contribute to painful intercourse. The lack of lubrication and support for the vaginal walls can reduce arousal during sex and increase friction, which in turn may produce soreness, burning, or irritation. Regular intercourse improves the muscle tone and lubrication of the vagina, so try not to avoid intercourse altogether. Masturbating regularly can also help you become aroused more easily and achieve orgasm.

SIMPLE SOLUTIONS TO GET STARTED
One way to combat vaginal dryness is to boost your water intake. Consume at least eight to ten eight-ounce glasses of water a day. This step is simple yet surprisingly helpful. Also, many personal bathing and laundry products contain perfume and other chemicals that can irritate the delicate mucosal tissues that line the vagina. It is therefore imperative to review the list of ingredients in such products before using them. A superfatty hypoallergenic soap with no dyes or fragrances and one that is nonalkaline is recommended.

ESTROGEN AND VAGINAL DRYNESS

If the problem is hormonal, estrogen may help. It can be taken as a tablet, applied vaginally as a cream, or inserted in a ring. This should help with vaginal dryness and pain during sex, but it's not going to boost your desire level—though if sex feels better, you may want to have it more often! Vaginal estrogen won't give you the systemic effects you'd experience when taking oral or patch estrogen. Also, risks and uncertainties surrounding its use are unknown.

I tried the cream and didn't love it. I found it was messy, a hassle, and didn't work particularly well for me. Using the ring is better for me. The only hard part is remembering to write on the calendar the date it is inserted; it has improved the quality of my life 100 percent. No more irritation—running to the bathroom all day and all night, etc. I never feel it—even in those intimate moments—and it does not slip. You can also take it out if you are worried, and reinsert it later.

The only thing I've had to consider is that although it is a local estrogen that is not supposed to increase my systemic levels of estrogen, it has actually done so. I was on the .075 patch when I first got the ring, and my doctor had to lower me to the .0375. I was just getting too much estrogen overall. The doctor says that occasionally she will see a patient who is affected systemically by Estring even though it isn't designed to do that.

—Tina

Side effects may include vaginal discomfort, abdominal pain, back pain, headache, genital itching, or leg swelling. Also, because the estrogen delivery is localized, very little estrogen is absorbed into the bloodstream, so it shouldn't interfere with other medications or treatments.

COMPLEMENTARY AND ALTERNATIVE TREATMENTS

Vitamin E supplementation has been shown to relieve some sexual problems, such as vaginal dryness or itching. You can start taking 400 IU of vitamin E every day for two weeks. If you see an improvement, you can increase the dosage to a total of 1,000 IU. It can also be taken as a vaginal suppository. Aside from taking vitamin E supplements, you can eat foods that are abundant in this vitamin. Avocado, wheat germ, flaxseed, and nuts are some examples of vitamin E–rich foods. Just adding a few nuts to your salad or avocado slices to your taco can make a difference.

LUBRICATION

I know lubricants are supposed to help, I do. But it's overwhelming to stand in the drugstore and look at six or seven different options and I have no idea which to choose. I don't know the difference, I just want one that will work for me!

—Kim

Lubrication is at the core of good feelings in sexuality. The use of a natural lube or massage oil can help wake up those sensual feelings. Any part of your body that is oiled, wet, slick, and smooth feels sexier than the same body part dry. "Remember, lubricants are only a penetration device," says the sex educator Wendy Strgar. "Even with the best lube in the world, if you aren't ready for someone to be inside of you, it isn't going to work. Lubricants should be used at the last minute, when you are aroused and excited and can't wait any longer."

There are several different types of lubricants. Water-based lubricants are by far the most popular category, often recommended by physicians and are latex-compatible. However, because of their ingredient base, which is largely petrochemical, some women may experience irritation, burning, and infection with use. Propylene glycol, a primary derivative used in antifreeze and brake fluid; polyethylene glycol, an ingredient of oven cleaner; and the preservatives methyl and propyl paraben are very common in water-based lube. The Campaign for Safe Cosmetics, a research advocate arm of the Breast Cancer Fund, has recently identified parabens as potentially carcinogenic and is working to stop their usage in all personal care products.

Another common ingredient of water-based lubricants is vegetable glycerin. This ingredient is a great antibacterial agent and does provide a certain glide, but in large amounts, it can potentially inflame yeast problems and feels very sticky and tastes overly sweet.

Many lubricant aficionados swear by silicone-based lubricants, known for providing a smooth and long-lasting glide. It is important to take into account potential health risks and the fact that it does not wash off very easily from sensitive tissue with soap and water. In addition, silicone-based lubricants may react chemically with some silicone toys, so the two shouldn't be used together.

There are a handful of companies that produce all-natural lubricants that are free of artificial ingredients and petrochemicals. Plus, they usually taste better! The women-owned and -operated Good Clean Love (www.goodcleanlove .com) is a small business with a great selection of these types of personal care products.

You've got the lubricant and you're ready to try it—now what? You may wish to experiment with several brands yourself before using with a partner. Find a quiet spot and enough time to play without interruption. Take some time to touch, smell, and taste each one so you are comfortable with it. Squeezing out some of the lubricant on your fingers and begin applying it to your vagina, starting with your vaginal lips. Pay plenty of attention to your clitoris and the surrounding area, massaging for several minutes.

Lubricants are best used to assist in foreplay. Foreplay is absolutely critical if adequate lubrication is a concern. Before intercourse, apply the lubricant to your vaginal opening or to your partner's penis. Men generally appreciate any extra attention given to their genitals.

Quick tip: Lubricants also come in handy to help with inserting tampons if you still occasionally have a menstrual cycle.

Avoid the use of petroleum-based lubricants such as Vaseline. Besides being thick, gooey, and messy, they weaken the latex in condoms. You may also be more likely to get vaginal infections as the goo helps hang on to bacteria that isn't meant to linger.

MOISTURIZERS

A personal lubricant is intended to provide temporary lubrication to reduce friction during sexual intercourse. While vaginal moisturizers make sexual intercourse more comfortable by restoring vaginal moisture, many women choose to add extra lubrication during sexual activity as well. Moisturizers such as Replens can also help if used regularly. Replens is estrogen-free and provides immediate relief for vaginal dryness. You can buy Replens in prefilled, disposable applicators or reusable applicators. This helps to rejuvenate the vaginal lining and eliminate dry skin cells and, when used regularly, replenishes your natural vaginal moisture. Moisturizers are long-lasting, so you have to apply them only every two to three days.

Other products come in a mousse form and may be easier to apply. Just shake the can well before use, hold it upside down, and dispense it directly onto your most private parts. (However, do not spray directly into the vagina). The personal lubricant mousse can be used all over the body.

Vaginal moisturizers are safe for oral sex and come in several different flavors. They are water-based and are safe for use with condoms.
They are not, however, a contraceptive, so plan accordingly. Until you
know how a certain product will work, panty liners are a must.

*I put it in at bedtime, and the next day is a little, er, juicy, but then things are
great. I have had the same experience as others, in that if you use this intermittently you get chunky discharge. I think it's because all the old cells build up and
can't get out. When I started using it every four days, the chunkiness stopped.
This has definitely made sex more comfortable, but also made me more comfortable just on a day-to-day basis.*

—Ellen

Some women may notice a discharge after the use of vaginal moisturizers; this is caused by the elimination of dead skin cells. Your body
naturally sheds dry vaginal tissue that has built up over time. A moisturizer helps this happen, leaving softer, more supple tissue behind.
When used on a regular basis, moisturizers will prevent the buildup of
dead skin cells, and the discharge should dissipate. If the discharge does
not dissipate, you may wish to wait an extra day or two between applications. Though use is recommended every two to three days, every
woman is unique, and you may wish to increase or decrease the amount
of time between applications to maximize moisture and minimize discharge.

WHAT TO AVOID

Stay away from highly perfumed bath products, as these will increase
vaginal dryness. Douching (cleansing your vagina with a liquid preparation) disrupts the normal chemical balance in your vagina and can
cause your vagina to feel dry or irritated. Most doctors and the American College of Obstetricians and Gynecologists (ACOG) suggest that
women steer clear of douching. All healthy vaginas contain some bacteria and other organisms called the vaginal flora. The normal acidity of
the vagina keeps the amount of bacteria down. But douching can change
this delicate balance. Upsetting that balance may make a woman more
prone to vaginal infections. Plus, douching can spread existing vaginal
infections up into the uterus, fallopian tubes, and ovaries. Bubble baths,
lotions, and anything similar can also cause irritation.

It's Not You, It's Me

If having intercourse is painful for you, your partner may be less willing to play, too. After all, he or she doesn't want to do anything that would hurt you. What if your partner isn't as interested as he or she used to be? There may be a few reasons:

- Your lack of lubrication may make sex uncomfortable for both of you.
- Your partner may be confused about what's happening with your body and not know if certain touches and techniques will still be pleasurable for you.
- If your partner is afraid your dryness means you're rejecting him or her, there may be the possibility of an altered sexual response, such as erectile dysfunction or great delay in reaching orgasm.
- Even if you give your partner the green light, having to watch you carefully for signs of pain may not create the best climate for hot sex!

Finding Pleasure

I used to be ready to go at a moment's notice; when our daughter was watching a movie, we'd sneak away for a few minutes. Not anymore. It just takes too long. It takes some of the spontaneity out of it, but now we know if we play around for ten or fifteen minutes first, then I'm good to go, and it's fun for me, too.

—Nora

Some women have fewer and less intense orgasms when their ovaries' function begins to diminish. It may take more time and stimulation to become aroused. But you can absolutely increase your likelihood of achieving satisfying sex. First, don't set yourself up with the expectation that you *must* have an orgasm. Instead, satisfying sex ought to have two goals: intimacy with your partner and pleasurable physical feelings.

I am twenty-seven and also have no libido, but to help me, my husband has bought me a small vibrator (the pocket rocket) . . . I know, but it really helps, and I orgasm every time we have sex. It definitely makes it more enjoyable. This method may not be for everyone!

—Kate

Taking matters into your own hands may prove to be helpful as well. Vibrators are sex toys that come in a wide variety of sizes, shapes, colors, and models (clit, G-spot, or remote control), also called dildos. The popular TV show *Sex and the City* made famous the Jack Rabbit vibrator, which features rotating beads, several speeds, and a clitoral stimulator. Walking into the average sex shop can be intimidating for some women, but there are a number of reputable online sites that cater to women, including:

www.goodcleanlove.com
www.adameve.com
www.mypleasure.com
www.blissable.com

Creating Intimacy

It's hard for me to feel sexy anymore. I think that's the hardest part for my husband to understand. I gain weight very easily on HT, and this makes me feel very self-conscious. My husband doesn't get how this upsets me and will tell me I'm beautiful at some of the moments I most need to hear it and least feel it myself. Just hearing these little words of encouragement have kept me going on some very challenging days.

—Sara

Sexuality is a delicate balance of emotional and physical issues. When women reject their partner's advances frequently, they may feel guilty. They feel they are disappointing their partners and fear serious damage to the relationship. Our emotional connections influence and are influenced by our physical connections. "I would say that it is through the physical conversations that I connect with my husband in ways that words cannot." This connection is where sex is making love. The more you love your partner, the more loving they become. There are several things you can do to keep an active sexual life. "It can become easy to focus on what isn't working perfectly in your sexual life," explains the sex educator Wendy Strgar. "Identifying with your sexuality instead of your dysfunction is the first critical step in reclaiming a healthy and satisfying sex life. Being awake to sexuality around you is a part of experiencing sensuality as a part of your nature."

Touching and intimacy often become more important than the physical pleasure of sex. This need to touch and be touched, physically and emotionally, is well worth nurturing. Such contact offers reassurance and comfort and the opportunity to show tenderness, companionship, and love. Make your partner a high priority. Pay attention to his or her needs and wants. Take time to understand the changes you both are facing. Try different positions; many women report that being on top feels more pleasurable. It may be that simply changing old habits can help increase your interest.

SEXUAL SUCCESS

According to research by Dr. James Kann, women with ovarian insufficiency and premature menopause have better sex lives if they:

- Work toward fulfillment of life goals
- Develop effective coping strategies
- Maintain a social/professional role
- Create a support network (family, friends, colleagues, and self-help groups)
- Receive quality medical care
- Seek many ways to create intimacy in relationship
- Have sexual self-confidence

Lesbian Sexual Intimacy

Many homosexual couples are familiar with the term "lesbian bed death," a phrase coined by the sociologist Pepper Schwartz in her 1983 book, *American Couples.* The phrase referred to the fact that lesbians report having less sex than any other type of couple after a few years together. If either partner is coping with hormonal issues, that may be playing a role.

Meanwhile, create more opportunities for intimacy. Talk, massage, play, or consult a sex guide like Felice Newman's *The Whole Lesbian Sex Book: A Guide for the Rest of Us,* which offers plenty of suggestions for creative physical intimacy, including a chapter that focuses exclusively on breast play. In fact, this would be a handy guide for anyone interested in expanding his or her sexual repertoire!

Successful Sexual Intimacy

Now more than ever, you need to communicate with your partner about what feels good and what doesn't. Try pleasure swapping. It sounds just like what it is: one night, your partner turns you on without you reciprocating; the next night, you do the same for your partner. This allows each partner to focus. The key is to tune in to what you want as well as respond to your partner's specific desires. Orgasm isn't mandated. Neither is intercourse. Again, it is about giving and receiving pleasure. One night you could request an erotic full-body massage. The next night it could be oral sex and no penetration. It is, again, about what feels satisfying for that particular person during that particular encounter. It's not about the same old "one-size-fits-all" approach to sex. It's about establishing new patterns of erotic behavior.

Eroticize each other's bodies instead of viewing sex just as a means to an end. In fact, one of the key exercises assigned to couples in sex therapy is the sensate focus technique, a practice of giving each other pleasure without intercourse. The relationship expert Dr. Les Parrott suggests, "This encourages couples to find creative ways to turn each other on. They rediscover each other's bodies and get back in touch with their sensuality, not just their sexuality. It gets them out of the cause-and-effect sexual routine. It's about tuning in to each other and in to real pleasure in new ways."

Get creative. Generate anticipation between the two of you for your "sex appointments." Actually, the excitement that can build up when you have a set sex date can be pretty hot. Tease and titillate each other. Discuss some of the things you're planning to do to each other. Prepare for the date the way you did at the beginning of your relationship. Wear something special. Set the scene. Intimacy dates can get you on the same page. They can foster a real sense of togetherness, open the door to more romance and flirting, and even lessen pressure and arguments over differing expectations. Book one tonight!

Take responsibility for your own needs and feelings. Work *together* to change what isn't working. Strive to approach each other in ways that will enhance the pleasure, reduce anxiety, and eliminate demand. Intimacy may take on an entirely new dimension. Learn to touch, hold hands, experiment, be together, and simply try to relax. You may rediscover yourself—and romance and sex—in very different and fulfilling ways.

Medications to Boost Your Sex Drive

Is there a female Viagra? Not yet. There are currently no FDA-approved treatments for women with low libido. Part of the problem is that for women, it's hard to pinpoint the exact problem. It might be your hormones, but it might not. "Yes, hormones matter, and in some women they can make some difference, but our sexuality is a many-splendored thing, and when something goes wrong you can't say it's only hormones, or it's only self-image, or it's only the relationship. For women it's always a combination of factors, and a simple Viagra-like solution will never be the answer for us," says Dr. Judith Reichman, an OB/GYN at Cedars-Sinai Medical Center in Los Angeles.

DHEA and l-arginine Amino Acid Cream

There are limited data suggesting that DHEA, and, to a lesser degree, l-arginine, may boost libido. However, we know little about their long-term safety, and recent studies don't necessarily qualify as being the most rigorous.

TESTOSTERONE SUPPLEMENTATION

Testosterone supplementation is the most widely used therapy but still sketchy in terms of research. Some women with high libido have low testosterone, and some women with low libido have high testosterone. Dr. Valerie Baker says, "In my personal experience, prescribing it for patients has not shown much help. If women take a lot—enough to raise serum testosterone a lot—then it may improve libido. The data about testosterone improving libido are best for higher doses of testosterone in women who have undergone removal of their ovaries." Anecdotal evidence seems to indicate it helps some women, too.

> *I used it nightly at first, then about every other night, then maybe twice a week. Now I rarely need to use it at all. My doctor told me when I started it that it would take two to four weeks to notice a difference in libido. It was two weeks exactly for me, although I did notice increased energy much sooner than that.*
>
> —Stephanie

Your insurance probably won't pay for it, and a $40 jar lasts about a month, but if it works, it may be well worth the investment. If testosterone is used at too high a level over a period of time, the side effects can be lingering or permanent. The side effects are hirsutism (male-pattern hairiness), facial oiliness, acne, deepening voice, hostility, weight gain, male-pattern baldness, elevated liver functions, and lower high-density lipoprotein (HDL). In any case, make sure you talk to your health care provider about both the pros and cons of testosterone supplements.

TYPES OF TESTOSTERONE

Testosterone supplements come in prescription injections, tablets, patches, gels, and creams. Most gels and creams on the market don't have specific approval for use in women, but some women use the gels or creams prescribed for men, in smaller amounts. Each formulation has benefits and risks in terms of cost, ease of application, and its ability to maintain consistent testosterone levels in your body over time. Replacement options include:

- **Oral:** Low-dose testosterone pills. Oral testosterone is processed through your liver and should not be taken if you have elevated liver enzymes, liver complications, or gallbladder disease.
- **Intramuscular:** Injections are rarely used in women, but are given twice a month. Testosterone levels are highest when you first inject, then fall over time. As seen in men, long-term use of injections may cause changes in your body's ability to make testosterone.
- **Topical:** Gels, creams, and patches are also available. Like small Band-Aids that you apply directly to your skin, they have to be changed often—every day to every few days. While they deliver consistent testosterone levels to your bloodstream, they are not available in a range of doses. With creams, your provider can set the dose to control the precise amount of hormone you receive.

As much fun as those nasty little side effects sound (and really, who wouldn't want to add some hostility and weight gain to the mix?), the best way to prevent undesirable testosterone side effects is to start out on a low dose.

If you'd rather apply a cream, low-dose creams are usually gentle and adjustable. Additionally, ask your doctor to measure your blood levels of testosterone about twelve hours after a dose, and try to keep your serum total testosterone level in the range of 40 to 50 ng/ml.

HOW TO APPLY TESTOSTERONE CREAM

Where you use it is up to you, but don't apply the cream in the same place every day. You can apply it to your:

- Wrists
- Abdomen
- Chest
- Under biceps
- Upper shoulders
- Neck
- Behind knees
- Buttocks
- Inner thighs
- Genital area

Do *not* use it on your breasts.

Women who overdo the testosterone cream can develop a condition called clitoromegaly (enlargement of the clitoris). Some women would consider that a problem; others would not. An enlarged clitoris may increase sexual sensitivity. If you are not using estrogen, you may find that it takes you a little longer to get results since your body may want to convert some of the testosterone to estrogen.

TOP WAYS TO BOOST YOUR SEX LIFE

- Get regular exercise—helps blood flow everywhere!
- Strive for eight hours of good sleep.
- Eat a balanced diet—you'll feel better.
- Smoking lowers your libido, so quit.
- Cut down or limit alcohol use.
- Do Kegels.
- Talk to your doctor about medications that may be interfering.
- Be in a mutually rewarding, healthy relationship.
- Get creative—everything from atmosphere to attitude play a role!
- Lose weight—we know it's hard, but a ten-pound weight loss can boost libido by 20 percent!

15

Adolescents' Needs

I was fourteen years old. And short. And flat-chested. It didn't bother me until my younger sister started her period and got taller than I was. She tried to hide it, but it seemed so unfair that she was growing and changing, and I had just stopped. I started stuffing my bras with tissues to make myself bigger, but I still felt like a freak.

The first doctor my mom took me to said I was just a "late bloomer" and did everything but pat me on my head and send us away. Luckily, my mother didn't give up and kept on trying until she found a doctor who would listen and actually do some tests. While we were glad to get some answers, we ended up with a lot more questions. Going through menopause in high school was not easy. At sixteen, I did go through puberty. However, I began having hot flashes, nightly sweats, mood swings, and sleepless nights, too. At least now we know what we're up against.

—Susanna

TO BE A MOTHER WATCHING her young daughter face a diagnosis with an implication beyond her understanding is heartbreaking. Yet a mother's attitude can play a significant role in how a young woman processes the diagnosis. Sometimes a mother's grief seems to overshadow her daughter's feelings. This can be true for several reasons. If the problem is hereditary or genetic in origin, then Mom may feel some guilt for passing along "faulty" genes. She may also mourn the loss of potential grandchildren and worry about long-term health implications. Unfortunately, too often a mom copes by withdrawing from her daughter.

When a young woman's mom cannot cope with the condition effectively, the daughter is left feeling even more isolated. Layer after layer is yet to be revealed to this young, vulnerable being over the next decade and beyond, and as a mother, the role of adviser can feel overwhelming. How can you discern which feelings are about your daughter and which about you? Guilt, fear, sorrow. Anger, helplessness, confusion. Yet that is just what we are called upon to do as mothers. Our daughters need us.

Symptoms in Adolescence

Girls with POI may have one or more of the following symptoms:

- Lack of breast development during puberty
- Lack of menstrual periods
- Decrease in breast size
- Hot flashes
- Vaginal dryness
- Mood swings
- Insomnia
- Slow growth in height or short stature

Not Getting a First Period

Today, many girls get their periods sometime between ages eight and thirteen, with the average age being more along the lines of twelve or thirteen. For teenagers who don't get their first periods, this is called primary amenorrhea. About 10 to 15 percent of girls with primary ovarian insufficiency never get a spontaneous first period. If a girl has normal secondary sex characteristics (including breast development and pubic hair) but still no first periods by the age of sixteen, she should seek medical care. Because the appearance of sex characteristics occurs about a year or two before the first period, if no secondary sex characteristics are noticed by age fourteen, a health care provider should be consulted at this time. With proper treatment, it is possible to induce the development of breasts and pubic hair as well as a period.

Irregular Periods

Many people just assume that it is normal for a teen's period to be irregular and sporadic. This is not the case. While a girl's body may not follow a 28-day cycle exactly, she should be somewhat consistent. Overall, a "normal" period for a teenager should look something like this:

- The average cycle length (from the first day of one period to the first day of the next) for a teen is between 21 and 45 days.
- Menstrual flow is between 2 and 7 days.
- Approximately 3 to 6 pads or tampons are used per day during a period.
- Period-related symptoms, while annoying, should not be debilitating or interfere with everyday life.

Anything outside these parameters could indicate problems and should be assessed by a health care provider. Hormone imbalances could be playing a role in cycle irregularity. This can include POI or polycystic ovary syndrome (PCOS). In addition, endocrine tumors or disorders of the thyroid gland can cause menstrual irregularities if the levels of the hormones in the blood become too low or too high. An event such as an illness or rapid weight changes, an eating disorder such as bulimia or anorexia nervosa, drug use, intense exercise, or stress can also make a teen's cycles more unpredictable. In any case, it is important to discuss this with your health care provider in order to determine the root cause.

Also, you should seek medical assistance as soon as possible if you encounter any of the following with your teen:

- Her periods are irregular for more than two years
- There is a family history of hormone imbalances
- Either the teen or a parent is worried about it

Getting a Diagnosis

I remember my diagnosis like it happened yesterday. Here I was, an eighteen-year-old, being told that I would never be able to have a child or be a mother. Throughout my childhood, I loved playing with my dolls, hoping to one day have my own real-life child. However, these dreams were shattered. I felt numb, not knowing what to think. I went home that day overwhelmed by a feeling of depression.

—Laurie

Some parents believe that if their child is not going to attempt to get pregnant at fifteen or sixteen, there is little need to discover the underlying cause of irregular cycles. After all, since there isn't a cure and pregnancy isn't an immediate goal, then what purpose is there in undergoing medical tests and procedures?

"The reason we are so concerned about irregular menstrual cycles in teen girls is that they can be a warning sign of an underlying disturbance in hormonal balance. Given that adolescence is the period of peak bone development and that normal hormonal functioning is essential for healthy bone growth, we are especially worried that these girls may be setting themselves up for a host of health problems, including low bone density, stress fractures, and osteoporosis later in life," explains Dr. S. Bryn Austin, a public health researcher in the Department of Adolescent/Young Adult Medicine at Children's Hospital Boston.

It is also important to seek out a specialist who is trained in pediatric gynecology. These types of physicians will know how to properly test your daughter and will best understand her unique needs.

Causes in Teens

It seems that the more common causes of POI in adolescents include cytogenetic abnormalities involving the X chromosome, ovarian dysfunction occurring in association with other autoimmune endocrine disturbances, and chemotherapy and/or radiation therapy given for any of a number of malignancies.

Support

The single most important thing to me over the past nine years has been my mother's support, encouragement, positive thinking, and love. Without her, I'm not sure where I'd be. So just being able to provide that for me was a great place to start—even if she didn't have all of the answers to what we should do next.

—Hannah

If you have been diagnosed with insufficient ovaries, you may feel alone and different. It may help you to know that there are thousands of other young women who have POI as well. It may also help you feel better to know that doctors and scientists are doing research to learn more about POI. Your emotions are already affected by the fluctuating hormones in your body, and the reality of your condition impacts your emotions even more.

WHAT YOUR DAUGHTER WANTS TO KNOW

We all like to assume we know what our kids need to know. But often this is based on our own perceptions and biases. Depending on your daughter's emotional maturity, age, and physical development, she might have very different needs for information. Here are a few important points to discuss with her when the time is right:

1. **It is normal to feel upset when your body doesn't work the way it should.** Teens and young women diagnosed with POI may feel sad, angry, depressed, and have feelings of loss. It might be a great help for teens to talk with other teens in the same situation. It is important for them to know they are not alone.
2. **POI is not the same thing as menopause, and it is not your fault!** A diagnosis of POI can hit young women at the heart of their self-esteem—and many think they will never feel normal again. It is important to educate young women about the realities of POI. POI means that their ovarian function has declined, not stopped entirely. Neither they nor their bodies have failed.
3. **You are not your POI.** POI alters a teen's sense of personal identity. It is important not to let teens define themselves by POI. Watch for subtle changes in language, i.e., POI becomes MY POI, or she continuously sees herself as a "POI patient" instead of a young woman who just happens to have POI.
3. **POI is more than just fertility.** For young girls, especially in the eyes of their mothers, a sense of lost fertility may prevail. The reality is that there are many roads to becoming a parent, and they will get there if this is what they truly desire.
4. **Give yourself time.** Sometimes teens and their families may have to rearrange previous plans and goals, but with a healthy mind

and body, new dreams are laid down in place of the old, and slowly but surely life feels good again—sometimes even better.

5. **You are in control.** Because of the very nature of POI, young women are acutely vulnerable to a sense of losing control. Any approaches or techniques that increase teen's participating and choices in the situation, from the most concrete (scheduling appointments) to the most profound and abstract (treatment decisions) will increase their sense of mastery and esteem.

6. **Focus on the adolescent.** Let your daughter know that life is a paradox. It is full of surprises, yet we never expect the unexpected. During our life cycle, there are certain medical conditions that we mentally gear up to, such as natural menopause in women. Access to a plethora of information makes coping with the condition far easier. And then there are a few other disorders that we never expect to have—like POI. Lack of suitable information, an overwhelming sense of grief, and other painful emotions associated with its diagnosis can wreak havoc in a young woman's life.

Still, with proper education and support, teens can learn to cope effectively and begin to view their POI experience as one teen patient describes it: "Everyone has 'stuff' in their life, so POI is mine, and in the great big scheme of things, it could be a lot worse."

HOW MOTHERS CAN PROVIDE SUPPORT

My mother tried to talk to me about it, but she, along with the other female members of my family, just made things worse. They all got married and had children young, then gave up work to look after them, and they all said I would just have to have a career, etc., instead. They said that having kids wasn't the be-all and end-all; when I mentioned that if it wasn't, why had they all had them? The stock response was that "Well, that's just what you do." They said they were sure I'd meet someone who would love me and who wouldn't mind about it—implying that there was a possibility that this wouldn't happen. I know they meant well, but it just made matters worse. In the end I used to just say that I would talk about it with my future partner when the time came and I didn't want to talk about it now.

—Lydia

When a young woman is diagnosed with ovarian insufficiency, she is more likely to rely on family support, especially if she still lives at home and does not have a partner. Her family plays an important part in helping her through this time. "They need to see themselves reflected in our eyes as still being whole, lovable, healthy young women," explains Karin A. Clark. "They need to know absolutely we are there and still love them. And we need to acknowledge our own experience fully, albeit separately and with others who can support us outside the family, so that we can remain as present as we long to be for this girl we adore."

HOW FATHERS CAN PROVIDE SUPPORT

The importance of parental acknowledgement, support, and understanding isn't limited to Mom, either. Dads, it is very important that you be there and available for your daughter during this time in her life, too. Fathers are often kept at a distance and protected from the emotional process, as this matter is seen as very personal and intimate. Dad's role can be very significant, explains Clark. "This will be the first man in her life to learn of her issue, and he has a huge responsibility to teach her she is a whole, complete, delightful woman in his eyes. Not to mention what a great mom and adult she will be, no matter how she chooses to arrive at her family, career, and other future choices.

"She needs to see your caring and belief in her during this time. Don't for one minute think that this is a 'woman thing,' thus leaving you with no role. You are the man in her life right now, the man who will affirm her value at this pivotal crossroads in her identity as a woman. Obviously, you walk a fine and fragile line here. 'Hey, honey, you are still so sexy and feminine' is hardly appropriate. Instead, gentle, simple truth is the path to consider: 'I love you, honey. I am so sorry you are going through something so hard in your young life. But you know, you will always be perfect to me.' And over the years, reinforce that any partner she ends up with had better be good enough, and he will be so lucky to have her."

IMPACT ON RELATIONSHIPS

I never really told any of my friends. I told one who didn't know what to say to me, and the conversation was dropped, so I decided it was best not to bother, and if I'm completely honest about it, I did, and still do, feel almost ashamed about it, even though I know I haven't done anything wrong, it's still something I feel embarrassed about.

—Karen

Relationships with peers may be affected simply because the odds are that no one else in a girl's immediate circle is likely to have ever heard of POI, much less know someone else who has it. They may try to reassure her, but, based on their own limited knowledge, the comforting words often fall short.

PROFESSIONAL SUPPORT

Research indicates that teens will probably need additional professional mental health support. For example, in one study, groups of teenagers with Turner syndrome and POI scored significantly higher on the shyness scale, social anxiety scale, and the Center for Epidemiologic Studies–Depression Scale, and lower on the self-esteem scale than did controls. The study highlights the need for additional support for teenagers.

With regard to how to deal with teenage girls when they are diagnosed, I would say the key is "kid gloves"—it's a lot to take in at any age, but to have to understand and deal with before you are really an adult and have even thought about such things is too much. Counseling, I think, should be made compulsory—I wish I could have had help dealing with it back then.

—Annie

Talk to your child's physician about referrals for mental health professionals, or contact your local children's hospital. Children's hospitals often have mental health professionals on staff who work exclusively with children and teens and their families who are facing difficulties.

PART FIVE

Looking Ahead

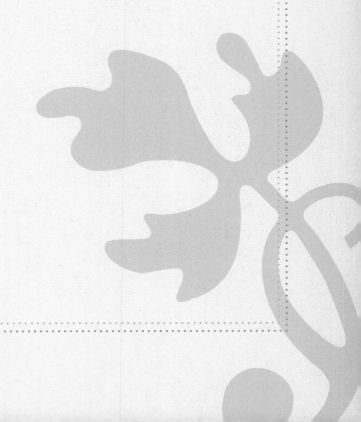

16

Planning Your Family

My experience with POI started when I was thirty-three, when my fiancé and I decided we wanted to have a baby. Within two months of that decision, my body started to show signs of POI. I started not having periods, and up until then my periods had always been very normal. At first I thought it might be the stress of working on having a baby, as I have always been a high-stress individual—so I figured I would focus on relaxing to see if that would change things. After a few months, I went to my doctor.

My doctor is a great guy; however, when it came down to telling me I had a problem, I read his diagnosis on the referral sheet to the fertility doctor—he never said a word. The sheet read that I should have an ultrasound to look at my ovaries due to ovarian failure. I sat for a good hour in his parking lot and cried. I was unaware of ovaries failing—I had it in my head that everyone my age could have a baby except for a very small amount of women. I have found that to be the total opposite! I had to deal with the fact that there wouldn't be any babies naturally, and that was very hard. I still believe we'll have little ones in our lives. I just don't know how that will happen yet.

—Laura

GROWING YOUR FAMILY MAY not be as easy as you had hoped. Even for those of us who describe ourselves as patient in other areas—babymaking is usually not one of them! For many women with ovarian insufficiency, getting pregnant may still be a possibility. And if you are unable to get pregnant, you may still be able to have children. Adoption or collaborative reproduction—becoming a parent with the help of egg donation and/or surrogacy—gives you more options and more hope than ever before.

Ovarian Insufficiency

Ovarian insufficiency may take away the possibility of becoming a mother for some women. "I wasn't sure if I even wanted children" and "I didn't know if I wanted more children" are commonly expressed feelings, but the frustration is that the decision has been taken away. A role that was longed for may not happen, at least not naturally or easily. How this feels and the impact it has will depend on individual circumstances, support networks and coping skills.

The Jean Hailes Foundation for Women's Health suggests that the important thing to do is to address the issue of roles and of purpose in your life. For example, if the mother role is important to you, what steps can you take to make this role a reality? Are donor eggs, foster care, or adoption options for you? Seek counseling to talk about the loss of this role if you need to, and if possible, include your partner (if applicable). It can also be helpful to ask what other roles you may have in your life and list those. Sometimes we have many roles, which we overlook when we get stuck wanting to fulfill one role and can't. Some women forget that they are also partners, daughters, sisters, friends, aunts, granddaughters, workers, neighbors, caregivers, and more.

Considering Pregnancy

Depending on each woman's unique circumstances, pursuing pregnancy may or may not be appropriate. Facilitating pregnancy in women with Turner syndrome is particularly dangerous, especially because such women have an increased risk of aortic rupture during pregnancy. "Even if an echocardiogram of the aortic root fails to show any dilatation, rupture may occur during pregnancy because the structure of the aortic wall is abnormal," explains Dr. Robert Rebar. "These data indicate that adoption is the more prudent course for individuals with gonadal dysgenesis, like Turner syndrome."

Getting Pregnant

Because many women with ovarian insufficiency do occasionally ovulate, it is possible to become pregnant without the assistance of a fertility doctor. In fact, about 5 to 10 percent of women with POI do become pregnant spontaneously. Usually, it's just a matter of luck. If you are fortunate enough to still be ovulating, timing sex is critical.

A woman's fertile "window" (days in the menstrual cycle when she can get pregnant) begins approximately five days prior to ovulation and lasts up to twenty-four hours after ovulation. This is because of the life span of the sperm, which remain viable in the woman's reproductive tract for up to five days, and the fact that the ovum can be fertilized for up to twenty-four hours following ovulation. However, the highest chances for conception are when you have sex within the two to four days before ovulation. Sex during this time period is most likely to result in a pregnancy.

Getting Professional Help

Most woman with ovarian insufficiency should schedule an evaluation with a fertility specialist or reproductive endocrinologist as soon as they want to become pregnant. You should do this even if you do not wish to become pregnant now, but think you may want to later. Because ovarian insufficiency can have detrimental effects on your fertility, you need to make fully informed decisions.

This is one time you need a specialist. Neither your primary care physician nor your OB/GYN is likely to have specialized training, and you need an expert. Too often, women are told to wait a year or two before testing because they are young, even though they have signs of ovarian insufficiency.

What to Expect at a Visit to a Fertility Doctor

Before your first visit, make sure previous fertility tests and other gynecological tests are sent to the specialist. If possible, take them ahead of time so your doctor can review the results. Include other medical results, such as diabetes or thyroid disease lab work.

You will need to answer tons of personal questions and complete a very thorough medical history. Then the doctor will do a comprehensive physical examination and pelvic ultrasound. More tests may be ordered, and a conversation will take place about your current and future family-planning goals.

QUESTIONS TO CONSIDER WHEN CHOOSING A REPRODUCTIVE ENDOCRINOLOGIST

How much does each assisted reproductive technology (ART) procedure cost? What is included in this cost?

What are your hours? How accessible is your clinic after hours?

Does the program meet and follow ASRM/SART guidelines?

Are one or more physicians board-certified in reproductive endocrinology?

What are the qualifications of the embryologist?

What types of counseling and support services are available?

Is donor sperm available in your program? Donor eggs? Donor embryos? Surrogacy?

Do you have an age or FSH cutoff?

What are your success rates for patients like me (i.e., similar in age, diagnosis, and medical history)?

How do you define "success"?

Who makes the final decision to cancel the cycle if my response to stimulation is suboptimal?

For a listing of fertility specialists and clinics, visit

- Society of Reproductive Endocrinology and Infertility at www.socrei.org
- Society for Assisted Reproductive Technology at www.sart.org
- CDC Art Report-www.cdc.gov/art

Tests and Procedures

OVARIAN RESERVE TESTING

It is important that any woman who has high FSH levels, POI, or signs of early menopause carefully assess her ovarian reserve before she embarks on any type of fertility treatments. Ovarian reserve testing looks at how many good-quality eggs you have left in your ovaries. For women with low ovarian reserve results, the chances of a successful pregnancy using her own eggs is low. Dr. Mark Perloe of Georgia Reproductive Specialists (GRS) explains, "When couples receive a diagnosis of poor ovarian reserve, it is also helpful for them to spend time talking with each other, examining their parenting needs. They might want to ask themselves, 'What is the most important thing to us about having a child? Is it the opportunity to provide love and support and guidance to a child? Is a genetic link essential? Is it important to experience pregnancy and childbirth? Can we look into adoption? Is child-free living a realistic alternative?' "

For more information about ovarian reserve testing, visit ReproSource, a leader in diagnostic testing for infertility, at www.reprosource.com.

How is your ovarian reserve assessed? While there are a number of tests available for evaluating ovarian reserve, there is some disagreement as to how these tests should be interpreted. Therefore it is important that you discuss all the results carefully with your doctor and consider all your options. Also, because age will continue to affect your reproductive potential, it is important to have your ovarian reserve checked periodically before pursuing any form of assisted reproductive technology. Each year we are learning more and more about ovarian reserve, what affects it, and how to measure it.

Most women start off by looking at their FSH and LH levels. Higher FSH levels are related to a decline in egg quality. Unfortunately, Dr. Perloe suggests, it is difficult to establish absolute values that define how high FSH levels can be and still achieve a pregnancy, especially due to variations in lab assessments and treatment options. Overall, it is not wise to rely on a single FSH value to fully assess ovarian reserve.

In addition to FSH, it is imperative to look at estradiol levels to gain insight into how the follicles are developing on the ovary. Values that are either too high or too low can indicate a problem with egg development. Progesterone levels should also be checked. A decline in ovarian reserve is sometimes associated with a short follicular phase (the time between when the egg is released and when your uterus is ready for the fertilized egg to implant or your period begins if you are not pregnant).

This contributes to a premature rise in progesterone levels, making the uterine environment less than ideal for the implantation of the fertilized egg.

Relatively new hormone tests include anti-Müllerian hormone (AMH) and inhibin B. Both of these hormones assist in the ovulation process. AMH is produced by the egg follicle and can indicate if your ovaries are still releasing eggs. AMH levels decrease as ovarian function begins to diminish. A normal range for AMH is usually over 1.0 ng/ml (however, too high an AMH level can indicate other ovarian problems, such as like polycystic ovary syndrome). If your AMH is under 0.6 ng/ml, this is a good indication that your ovarian function is insufficient and most likely you are not releasing very many good-quality eggs.

Inhibin B is another hormone produced by the ovaries. It works to inhibit FSH, which helps your follicles develop. As ovarian function diminishes, you produce less inhibin B, which causes FSH levels to rise and further impairs ovulation. Typically, a normal inhibin B level is anything above 45 pg/ml. While both of these tests are still considered investigational, there is more research being conducted about their importance in assessing ovarian reserve.

An antral follicle count is another test that can provide you with information about your egg reserve. Antral follicles (or resting follicles) are small follicles that can be seen using a vaginal ultrasound. The number of visible antral follicles is indicative of the number of other follicles remaining in the ovary. If there are only a few antral follicles visible, there are probably far fewer eggs remaining than if there are many visible follicles.

How many antral follicles are considered good? According to the Advanced Fertility Center of Chicago:

- Less than 4 is an extremely low count and indicates very poor or no response to stimulation.
- 4 to 7 is still considered a low count and there is still concern about a possible poor response to stimulation.
- 8 to 10 is a reduced count associated with a reduced chance of pregnancy.
- 11 to 14 is considered "normal," and stimulation is somewhat adequate.
- 15 to 30 is very good and should have an excellent response to ovarian stimulation.

- Over 30 is very high and may indicate a risk for PCOS or overstimulation if fertility medications are used.

REPEAT TESTING

Several methods have been developed to estimate the functional or biological age of the ovaries. Since ovarian reserve can vary over time, any results suggesting limited ovarian reserve should be confirmed by further testing in subsequent months. It may be that inflammatory, infectious, or autoimmune conditions are contributing to the abnormal results. Any potentially reversible causes of diminished ovarian function should be corrected, particularly in younger women.

Treatment Options

There are a number of different fertility treatment options, ranging from inexpensive and easy to very expensive and extremely invasive. Some are more effective than others.

OVULATION INDUCTION

For many women trying to conceive, doctors will prescribe a medication to induce ovulation. Clomiphene citrate is often the first line of treatment for women who can't get pregnant. Unfortunately, it doesn't work well for women with POI. Dr. Valerie Baker, the medical director at the Stanford Fertility and Reproductive Medicine Center In Vitro Fertilization Clinic, explains, "Clomiphene is an antiestrogen or, more technically, a selective estrogen receptive modulator. It works well in women who already on their own make estradiol [estrogen] by blocking the estrogen receptor, making the woman's body think that there isn't much estrogen around. So then the pituitary gland increases its production of FSH and LH, and that in turn stimulates the ovary to ovulate.

"In women who have POI, they have low estradiol concentrations most of the time, and so there isn't much estrogen to block. In addition, women with POI already have high levels of FSH and LH; their body is already trying as hard as it can to stimulate the ovary to release an egg, but there aren't many or any eggs left in the ovary to release. For women with POI, there isn't a benefit of trying to raise the FSH and LH any higher."

IN VITRO FERTILIZATION (IVF)

With in vitro fertilization (IVF), a woman is given large doses of hormones to stimulate the development of healthy egg(s) in the ovaries. Eggs are then surgically removed from the ovaries and mixed with sperm outside the body in a petri dish (*in vitro* is Latin for "in glass"). As specified by the American Society of Reproductive Medicine (ASRM), after about forty hours, the eggs are examined to see if they have become fertilized by the sperm and are dividing into cells. These fertilized eggs (embryos) are then placed in the woman's uterus, bypassing the fallopian tubes.

The problem with IVF is that it works well for many fertility problems, but most IVF cycles use FSH to stimulate a woman's ovaries to produce more than one egg for that cycle. If you have a low ovarian reserve and high FSH, giving you more FSH doesn't necessarily do anything; the ovary doesn't necessarily respond any better—in fact it seems it usually doesn't. Most reproductive endocrinologists consider a day 3 FSH value over 10 to be too high for comfort in order to start IVF.

LOW-STIMULATION IVF

Low-stimulation IVF may be a better option for women with a low remaining ovarian reserve. Low-stimulation IVF simply reduces the high levels of fertility medication used in traditional IVF. As Dr. Sherman Silber of the Infertility Center of St. Louis explains, women with low remaining ovarian reserve "normally yield very few eggs anyway even with huge megadoses of gonadotropins. If they have any quality eggs remaining, low stimulation is just as likely to yield as many eggs (very few, of course) as giving huge megadoses of gonadotropins. Even in the worst-case scenario, if there are no good eggs left at all, at least they can discover this with only $400 spent on drugs instead of $7,000, the cost of maximum dosage."

Dr. Silber continues, "Think of this simple parable: If you are sitting under an apple tree and wish to eat the most ripe and ready apples, you have a choice. You can chop down the tree and look at every apple on the fallen tree to see which ones were ready. Or you can simply try to shake the lower branches and eat the one or two that have fallen. That is the idea of mini-IVF. It may not work for everyone, but for many patients, it will remove much of the aggravation and complexity associated with IVF and also dramatically reduce the cost. It is an ingeniously conceived and completely different approach to IVF, which saves the patient much of the complexity and cost associated with more conventional IVF protocols."

Third-party Reproduction

Third-party reproduction involves using an egg or embryo donor, a sperm donor, and/or a surrogate. There are significant emotional, physical, financial, and moral concerns involved in making such a decision, and accessing the best professional resources available can help you make the right decision for your particular situation.

EGG DONATION

I decided as soon as I was diagnosed as going through early menopause that I would investigate using donor eggs. This took some of the pressure off. Of course I would have liked my own genetically born children, but if that is not to be, then I'll be damned if I'm going to miss out on being a mother.

—Barbara

Women who have diminished ovarian function and are unable to produce good-quality eggs or lack eggs altogether may be good candidates for egg donation. A form of collaborative reproduction, egg donation is the process by which a woman (the egg donor) provides eggs to another woman (the recipient) for purposes of assisted reproduction. First, the donor's ovaries are stimulated by fertility drugs to produce extra eggs. These eggs are then retrieved from the donor and fertilized with the male partner's (or donor) sperm in the laboratory. The resulting embryos are transferred back to the recipient's uterus. If a pregnancy occurs, the recipient will be able to carry the pregnancy and give birth. She will have a biological connection, but not a genetic relationship to the child; her partner will be both biologically and genetically related if his sperm was used.

The first pregnancy achieved with egg donation was performed in 1983. Since that time, thousands of babies have been born through egg donation. In fact, today, more than ten thousand families choose to use donor eggs each year. Egg donation has a relatively high success rate, with nearly half of all egg donation cycles resulting in a pregnancy.

FINDING AN EGG DONOR

I had to look at about a hundred-plus donors before I found someone I liked. It's a major freak-out and sooo abnormal finding part of the genetic makeup of your child, as if you were shopping for a used car. It took me a long time to get past that! If you stick it out, you will eventually find the right donor.

—Rebecca

There are several ways to locate egg donors. You can talk to your fertility clinic, an independent egg donation agency, or even a reproductive attorney about helping you find an appropriate donor who will be a good match for your family. In general, the donor must be a healthy nonsmoker who is twenty-one to thirty-two years old. She should also undergo extensive medical, psychological, and genetic testing, as well as screening for infectious diseases, such as HIV and other sexually transmitted infections.

Egg donors can be anonymous or known to you (like a friend, sister, or cousin). Most commonly, egg donors are anonymous and known only to the couple through a photo and profile page. Couples often feel more secure in knowing that their anonymous egg donor will not be involved in the pregnancy. A known donor is someone whom the woman wishing to become pregnant knows—a relative, a friend, or acquaintance. Depending on the egg donor agency or clinic, a woman who is previously unknown to the couple may meet and get to know them. The advantage of using a known donor is that more information is available about their medical and personal histories.

In any case, comprehensive physical and psychological screenings are important parts of the process, as well as counseling for both parties. Almost all egg donors indicate that a primary motivating factor was a desire to help someone else build a family. Many donors have children of their own and want to share that opportunity. For some donors, there can be a financial incentive as well. Donors are typically paid about $7,000 for their time and effort. This amount may be slightly higher when donors are chosen for very specific criteria that may be difficult to find, such as a particular ethnic group, or very high academic or athletic standards.

Depending on you and your partner's wishes, discuss the qualities you're looking for, including:

- body height and build
- eye and hair color
- blood type
- ethnic background
- religious background
- occupation
- level of education
- academic achievements
- special interests

No matter which egg donor you choose, above all else, work with an ethical clinic or agency. This includes ensuring the physical and emotional well-being of you and your donor, both now and in the future. Egg donation will forever be a part of your family history. It is important to go into this as prepared as possible so you can not only reap the rewards of this wonderful family building option but also be able to deal effectively with any issues that may arise.

SURROGACY

In a surrogate pregnancy, the couple chooses to have another woman gestate the embryos they create. Surrogacy is a complex and expensive endeavor, but it is sometimes the only option for some couples. As with any type of collaborative reproduction, you are going to want to do your homework. Start with checking out the surrogacy laws in your home state. If you live in a state that is not surrogacy-friendly, you might need to seek out surrogacy in another state. Also, talk with others about their surrogacy experiences and any resources they recommend. The surrogacy arrangement involves an attorney and can be made through an independent agency or contracted privately. While some families opt to find their surrogate on their own, a surrogacy agency can provide a lot of valuable assistance and resources making the process much easier. For example, a good agency should be able to:

- Properly screen all surrogates in terms of physical and emotional health and overall well-being
- Match you with a surrogate with whom you are comfortable

- Provide you with assistance in finding the proper insurance coverage for your surrogate throughout her pregnancy
- Provide the legal support in terms of paperwork, contracts, payments, and a pre-birth order
- Ensure that the surrogate attends all medical appointments and receives any necessary medical care
- Provide ongoing support to both surrogate and recipient families

There are two major types of surrogates: gestational and traditional. In a gestational surrogacy, the intended parents create embryos that are transferred to the surrogate mother via IVF. The surrogate mother gestates the child but has no genetic link to the child. The eggs can be provided by either the intended mother or by an egg donor. The legal steps to confirm parentage with the intended parents are generally easier with gestational surrogates than in traditional surrogacy because there is no genetic connection between the child and surrogate.

With a traditional surrogacy arrangement, the surrogate mother donates her own egg as well as her uterus. The recipient partner or a donor provides the sperm that is used to fertilize the egg though intrauterine insemination (sometimes called artificial insemination). The surrogate mother gestates the embryo and has a genetic link to the child.

Generally, a woman must meet the following criteria to be considered a good candidate for becoming a surrogate mother.

- Between twenty-one and thirty-eight years of age
- Given birth to one or more children previously, with no complications
- No history of sexually transmitted diseases
- In good health, with no chronic medical conditions
- Average weight for her height
- A nonsmoker who lives in a smoke-free home
- No illegal drug use
- Exhibits emotional stability

Surrogacy is a medically and emotionally complex process involving medical, mental health, and legal professionals all working together to ensure the procedure is successful for both the surrogate and the intended parents.

EMBRYO DONATION

Using someone else's previously created embryos may be another way to build your family. After an IVF cycle, embryos can be frozen (or cryo-preserved) for later use. If the previous IVF cycle is successful, particularly if the pregnancy resulted in multiples, the biological parents of the embryos may decide to donate their leftover embryos to someone else.

A fertility clinic may have embryos that couples have released for donation. Some agencies match donor and recipient couples, and others have identified themselves as embryo "adoption" agencies, even though there is no such legal term. Only a child who has been born can be placed for adoption. However, these agencies, which are typically expensive, operate in a similar fashion as a traditional adoption agency, including a thorough home study.

SCREENING Embryo donation requires that the recipient couple undergo the appropriate medical and psychological screening recommended for all gamete donor procedures. In addition, the female partner undergoes an evaluation of her uterine cavity and then her endometrium is prepared with estrogen and progesterone in anticipation of an embryo transfer.

In the United States, embryo donation must meet established FDA guidelines for screening of the donors. In the case of embryos that have been created previously, the FDA recommends, but does not require, that the couple who created these embryos undergo the requisite screening and testing required of all egg and sperm donors. For embryos that are created specifically for donation, the sperm donor and egg donor must be screened and tested like any other sperm and egg donors who are not intimate sexual partners of the recipients.

ETHICAL ISSUES SURROUNDING EMBRYO DONATION Embryo donation is a controversial process from both the ethical and legal standpoints. What differentiates embryo donation from either egg or sperm donation is that the child born to the couple will have no genetic link with either parent. Of paramount importance is that informed consent and counseling be provided to both the donors of the embryos and the recipient couple to address all of the potential issues embryo donation may raise. In addition, due to the absence of explicit laws regarding embryo donation, couples should seek legal counsel regarding the necessity of a predonation agreement as well as a judicial determination or recognition of parentage.

SUCCESS RATES FOR FROZEN EMBRYOS Success rates of embryo donation are difficult to assess and depend on the quality of the embryos that were frozen, the skill of the embryologist who froze the embryos, the age of the woman who provided the eggs, her fertility diagnosis, and the number of embryos transferred. There are no national statistics on the success of embryo donation due to the limited number of embryo donation cases nationwide.

Adoption

> There are options for people with ovarian insufficiency, including adoption, which I very strongly support and hope to be able to do one day. There are many children out there looking for loving homes and parents. One thing I used to torment myself with is "I won't be able to pass my genetic material on to anyone— no one will be able to say 'Wow, your daughter has your eyes.' " But the more I thought about it, those aren't the things that count. And my adopted children will *have* similarities to me—their learned behaviors. So all those annoying, obnoxious things I do will *be passed on after all!*
>
> —Dee

Adoption is another option for family building. As Dawn Davenport, the author of *The Complete Book of International Adoption: A Step-by-Step Guide to Finding Your Child,* points out, there isn't one right way to build your family. Infertility treatment is not superior to adoption nor is adoption a cure for infertility. "Adoption isn't more noble than sticking with assisted reproductive technology. Using your own eggs with IVF is not necessarily better than using donor eggs. Domestic adoption is not superior to international adoption, and vice versa. Adopting from Ethiopia is great, but there are great kids in Louisiana, Thailand, New York, Taiwan, and California as well. Foster care adoption is a wonderful way to add a child to your family, but it's not for everyone."

There are a number of different options for adding to your family through adoption:

- **International adoption.** A number of countries will allow couples to adopt children from their orphanages. In most cases, international adoptions are finalized in the country of origin, so once you come home with your child, he or she is already legally yours. There are a number of countries that work with U.S. couples hoping to adopt, so identifying which country works best for your family is usually the first step you should take.
- **Domestic adoption.** A domestic adoption is when you adopt a child from the country in which you live. Adoption laws vary widely from state to state. You may adopt a child who is in the foster care system or an infant, either independently or through an agency or facilitator.

TYPES OF ADOPTION PLANS

- **Open adoption.** The birth parents specify the type of family they would consider most appropriate as a placement for their child. They meet the chosen family prior to placement, and identifying information is shared by both parties. An open adoption is considered a lifelong relationship with ongoing contact over the years, such as attending the birth of the child, attending physician visits together, visiting the home, gathering as extended family members on special occasions, and others.
- **Semiopen adoption.** An agency or third party mediates the contact between the parties before and after the birth. In semiopen adoption, the birth parents may specify particular characteristics with regard to the adoptive family. The birth parents may also meet the adoptive parents either before delivery or after placement on a first-name basis. After placement, the birth parents may receive pictures and letters from the adoptive family through the agency.
- **Closed or confidential adoption.** A closed adoption is one in which the birth parents have little or no control over the placement of their child. The adoptive family receives information about the birth family's medical history up to the point of placement. There is no planned, ongoing sharing of social and medical information after the adoption is finalized. Access to finding a

birth parent is limited by law and must be by mutual agreement at the time the child is of legal age. The adult child must contact the state central adoption registry.

CHOOSING ADOPTION PARTNERS

Choosing an agency or adoption attorney to help you through the process is one of the most important choices you will have to make. Start with a lawyer, choosing one that is a member of the American Academy of Adoption Attorneys (AAAA or Quad A), a professional membership organization with standards of ethical practice. Adoption law is typically state-specific except for a few federal laws, so you want an adoption attorney that is well versed in the adoption laws of your state.

- **Independent adoptions** by attorneys are one of the most cost-effective ways to adopt. Attorneys must adhere to the standards of the Bar Association, and some attorneys who specialize in adoption are members of the American Academy of Adoption Attorneys.
- **Agency adoptions** provide the greatest assurance of monitoring and oversight since agencies are required to adhere to licensing and procedural standards.
- **Placements by adoption facilitators** offer the smallest amount of supervision and oversight. This does not mean that there are not ethical professionals with good standards of practice; it simply means there are few or no oversight mechanisms in place at this time. For some, this is the riskiest and most expensive way to adopt.

Preserving Your Fertility

FREEZING EGGS

Depending on how early you are diagnosed, freezing your eggs may be an option. Though freezing unfertilized eggs is still considered investigational, many advances have been made. Before you decide to freeze your eggs, talk to your doctor about the realistic chances for success. And go to a reputable clinic with significant experience with egg freezing. Even under the best of circumstances, egg freezing is not as successful as freezing embryos. There are still many unanswered questions about egg freezing: How long can eggs be frozen? How many eggs should be frozen? If you have cancer, how will egg freezing affect your treatments in terms of delaying them or in the hormones used?

Egg freezing may be an option for women who may not have a partner yet and want to preserve their eggs for later use. Again, egg freezing is expensive—about $15,000 to $20,000 to obtain and freeze the eggs plus another $15,000 to $20,000 for each IVF attempt. Storage fees rack up another $1,000 per year.

OVARY CRYOPRESERVATION

Thin slices of ovarian tissue can be recovered laparoscopically and successfully frozen in liquid nitrogen. The immature eggs contained in the ovary survive the freezing process better than do mature, ovulated eggs. Ovarian cryopreservation and subsequent reimplantation are important to women diagnosed with cancer, blood diseases, or other disorders that require radiation and chemotherapy, which can cause infertility. If they can have an ovary removed before the eggs are damaged, they might later be able to have biological children. A fairly new technique, this method requires surgery.

The goal is to preserve hundreds or even thousands of immature eggs within the ovarian tissue for later use. Because this eliminates the need for mature eggs, this procedure can be made available to much younger girls, even before they reach puberty. The major drawbacks include the highly experimental nature of the procedure and the fact that success has been limited. Also, there are many ethical concerns about girls' undergoing this type of complicated surgical procedure when they are too young to fully comprehend the implications and possible complications.

Adding to your family may be more difficult (and more expensive) than you dreamed of. "I like to say my kiddos just had a higher start-up cost than most," says Robin, a mom with POI who adopted two children. There are many resources available to help cover the expenses of adoption and fertility care, as well as professional consultants who can assist you in looking at the best options for your particular situation. For more information about family-building assistance, check the Resources section at the end of the book.

Birth Control—Are You Kidding Me?

> *The one advantage of being in premature menopause ought to be the end of periods. The truth is, there is no way to know when I will menstruate. The fluctuation is extraordinary. Am I ovulating? Who the hell knows? It ain't likely, as I only had one period last year, but anything's possible. If one egg makes it and there is one strong swimmer about, possibilities exist for babies. So what do we do?*

> —Anna

Even if you aren't likely to have a rogue egg flying down your tubes, as long as you have a uterus and at least one ovary, you can still get pregnant. If you have ovarian insufficiency, you are much more likely to have a random cycle. With POI, the younger you are, the more likely you are to have a cycle off and on. That's a general rule, so plan accordingly. Thus, barrier contraception may be warranted if pregnancy is not desired by sexually active women. Pregnancy has even occurred spontaneously at age forty-four in a patient diagnosed with premature ovarian failure at age twenty-eight. It doesn't happen often, but it does happen. In fact, about 5 to 10 percent of women with POI conceive spontaneously.

Birth control pills (BCPs) are a possibility if you do not want to become pregnant. Though they may be a good choice if vaginal dryness is an issue, there are two problems with BCPs: there is no estrogen during the placebo week and more estrogen than you need for replacement the rest of the month. The main issue with BCPs is that the hormone amounts are appropriate for women with "typical" hormone levels. For women with high FSH and low estrogen, BCPs or any other type of hormone contraceptive may not work as well to prevent pregnancy.

The sponge is still around, and so is the diaphragm. Spermicide is another possible alternative. With vaginal dryness already an issue, many women prefer not to use condoms (but should if they are not in a long-term monogamous relationship and want to avoid sexually transmitted diseases, as well as pregnancy). As with any choice, discuss this with your health care provider. Think carefully about your short- and long-term needs and pick an effective birth control option accordingly.

FMR1 TESTING

Women who have been diagnosed with primary ovarian insufficiency or premature ovarian failure should be tested for the FMR1 genetic premutation. Women with POI/POF are at higher risk for having a FMR1 genetic premutation compared to the general population. The FMR1 gene on the X chromosome, produces a protein called the FMR1 protein that is critical for intellectual development. Within this gene, there are repeating sequences of DNA known as CGG repeats. Every person has an FMR1 gene containing approximately 5 to 40 CGG repeats. Women with higher than normal CGG repeats have a greater risk of having children with fragile X syndrome, the most common cause of inherited mental impairment, ranging from learning disabilities to severe mental retardation including autism or "autistic-like" behavior. It is important to talk with your health care provider or genetic counselor about your individual risk and the need for further genetic testing.

17

A Lifetime of Living Well

At age fifty, it feels odd to be considered a long-term survivor of POI. But that is indeed what I am. To have been diagnosed at age twenty-nine, I have had twenty years of trial and error to discover what works best for me. But, boy did I feel isolated twenty-plus years ago, when the doctor told me of my diagnosis and that there was "nobody" to whom I could talk who had this condition because it was "extremely rare." Today I am more energetic, happier, more positive now than ever before. I do step aerobics, walk four miles a day, and study nutrition.

—Elaine

Creating a Lifelong Plan

Patients with ovarian insufficiency should be seen by a health care provider at least annually to monitor their HT. You should also get any other routine screenings done on schedule. For example, symptoms and signs of thyroid disease and adrenal insufficiency should be checked for during annual follow-up visits. TSH levels should be checked every three to five years (every year if the antiperoxidase antibody test is positive). Stress, pregnancy, breast feeding or other life changes may necessitate additional medical care. Preventing long-term health problems is important for everyone, but especially for women with ovarian insufficiency. Your hormone imbalance puts you at risk for some specific health issues, including cancer, heart disease, and bone loss.

The most important thing I learned is that I have to be CEO for my health care. Once I went off the hormones after breast cancer, my OB wasn't sure what to do with me. He's supernice, but he mostly just delivers babies. I was the one who reminded him it was time for my bone scan and that I should get a mammogram. I don't give up responsibility for taking care of my body anymore.

—Robin

Cancer

Many women are concerned that HT will give them a higher risk of breast cancer. The reality is that despite a number of scientific studies that have tried to prove a link between HT and breast cancer, the data are still somewhat contradictory. The studies appear to reveal that there may be a small increase in breast cancer risk for long-term (longer than eight years) users of HT. But the same studies also appear to show that women using HT have a lower risk of dying from breast cancer than women who develop breast cancer and haven't used HT. Don't forget—*none* of these studies has included younger women for whom HT is imperative, and whose needs and issues are completely different from those of older women.

More than half of all cancers are preventable by making lifestyle changes and getting regular medical checkups. Here are some tips from the American Cancer Society that can help save your life.

Tips for Preventing Cancer
- **Quit smoking.** Smoking damages nearly every organ in the human body, is linked to at least fifteen different cancers, and accounts for some 30 percent of all cancer deaths.
- **Stay out of the sun.** A mix of methods—finding shade; wearing hats, sunglasses, and protective clothing; and applying sunscreen—is needed to protect against skin cancer.
- **Limit alcohol consumption to no more than one drink a day.** Alcohol raises the risk of cancers of the mouth, pharynx (throat), larynx (voice box), esophagus, liver, and breast, and probably of the colon and rectum. People with a history of breast cancer should not drink.

- **Eat your fruits and veggies.** Studies suggest that people who eat more vegetables and fruits, which are rich sources of antioxidants, may have a lower risk of some types of cancer.
- **Watch your body mass index (BMI).** Obesity is linked with an increased risk of several types of cancer.
- **Move.** Engage in at least thirty minutes of moderate to vigorous physical activity, above your usual activities, on five or more days of the week; forty-five to sixty minutes of intentional physical activity are preferable.

CANCER SCREENING

You may already do a monthly breast exam and skin check and have Pap smears, but you may be missing other cancer screenings. Go to the American Cancer Society's Web site (www.cancer.org) and accept the Great American Health Challenge. Take the Health Check by answering some questions about yourself (or a loved one) and instantly get a personalized health action plan to share with your doctor.

Protect Your Heart

Heart disease is a serious health concern for women. Heart disease, or cardiovascular disease (CVD), claims the lives of more than 500,000 women each year. This is more than the next sixteen common causes of death in women combined, including all forms of cancer (including breast cancer). Though it is very rare for a young woman with POI to develop heart disease right away, certain factors related to the disorder might increase her chances of developing heart disease later in life.

- The lower levels of estrogen in POI can lead to higher levels of low-density lipoprotein (LDL) cholesterol. LDL is known as "bad" cholesterol because it is the main source of the buildup in and blockage of arteries that can lead to heart attacks.
- The lower levels of estrogen in POI can also lead to lower levels of high-density lipoprotein (HDL) cholesterol, known as "good" cholesterol because it helps prevent buildup in and blockage of the arteries.

- After some time, buildup of cholesterol in the arteries can cause "hardening of the arteries," which means that the blood flow to the heart is slowed down or blocked. Blood carries oxygen to the heart. If the heart can't get enough oxygen, a person may have chest pains. If the blood supply to part of the heart is cut off completely because of blockage, the result is a heart attack.

THE ROLE OF ESTROGEN

Getting adequate estrogen therapy may help guard against heart disease. Estrogen helps the body by:

- Keeping the lining of the arteries healthy
- Relaxing muscles that control arteries to allow better blood flow to tissues
- Normalizing LDL and HDL levels to decrease cholesterol buildup in the arteries that could lead to blockage

CHOLESTEROL

Many studies have found that women with higher total cholesterol levels also have higher rates of coronary artery disease. As ovarian function diminishes and hormone levels change, the development of atherosclerosis (a buildup of cholesterol in the coronary arteries) can progress. Left untreated, atherosclerosis can eventually cause a heart attack by blocking the supply of blood to the heart.

PROTECT YOUR HEART

For more information on heart health and to learn more about what you can do to stay healthy and watch for warning signs of heart attack, visit the American Heart Association's Web site at www.americanheart.org.

CONTROLLING RISK FACTORS Behavioral modification is extremely beneficial in controlling cardiovascular risk. Dietary restriction and physical activity are known to lower elevated cholesterol levels and decrease blood pressure. For women working to prevent CVD, some important guidelines to reduce risk include:

- **Know your family history.** Those with family members who have heart disease have a greater chance of experiencing the same. Knowing this may help you take steps to improve your health.
- **Quit smoking.** Women should consider smoking and secondhand smoke as a significant risk factor that can be avoided.
- **Control your blood pressure.** Evaluating and treating elevated blood pressure can positively impact the risk of CVD. Lifestyle modification—weight control, increased physical activity, alcohol intake moderation, and moderate sodium restriction—can be helpful in controlling blood pressure.
- **Reduce your cholesterol level.** Having your cholesterol level measured at least every five years may be beneficial. Interpreting HDL, LDL, and triglyceride levels should be done with every cholesterol result. The primary goal of LDL (bad cholesterol) management is to reduce it to less than 160 mg/dl in low-risk individuals and less than 130 mg/dl in higher-risk individuals. Your physician can help determine your risk and LDL goal.
- **Increase your physical activity.** At least thirty minutes of moderate-intensity activity (brisk walking, jogging, cycling, or other aerobic activity) most days of the week, as well as increased daily lifestyle activities, is encouraged. Regular exercise improves conditioning and promotes optimum fitness. Before starting any exercise program, discuss with your physician the types of exercise and goals to be set.
- **Control your weight.** Your doctor should assess your body mass index (BMI) by measuring your height and weight and compare with optimal values. Work to achieve the recommended BMI of between 18 and 25.
- **Control your diabetes.** Women with diabetes are at higher risk of CVD. Proper blood sugar control can help to decrease the risk of CVD.
- **Eat fish (or at least take fish oil).** Omega-3 fatty acids benefit the hearts of both healthy people and those at high risk of—or who have—cardiovascular disease. The American Heart Association

recommends eating fish (particularly fatty fish) at least twice a week.

- **Talk to your health care provider** about your risk for heart disease and determine which steps you can take to lower your risk.

SOY AND HEART DISEASE

Soy-rich foods reduce total cholesterol, bad (LDL) cholesterol, and triglyceride levels. The Food and Drug Administration (FDA) has approved soy dietary supplementation and states that including 25 grams of soy per day in a prudent diet may reduce the risk of heart disease.

Protect Your Bones

Bones, bones, bones. I would be happy if my doctor never mentioned the word again. It's the bone concern that keeps me awake at night wondering what to do for the best. That's the only thing that makes me consider HT. I feel pretty comfortable looking at alternative treatments for the rest of my symptoms, but I've seen what osteoporosis can do, and it scares me. I don't want to be the old lady who's all hunched over just because I was too damn stupid to take the hormones. But I haven't started yet.

—Liz

Osteoporosis is a bone disorder that decreases bone strength and increases the risk of breaks and fractures. Estrogen helps conserve calcium and other minerals in bones and protects against bone loss. POI can cause women to lose bone density or bone strength, one of the major factors leading to osteoporosis. While POI has been widely associated with lower bone mineral density and increased osteoporosis risk, its impact on fracture risk is not well quantified. Even though osteoporosis is more common in people age fifty and above, women with POI may develop the condition at a much younger age. An adequate level of estrogen in the body is an important factor in preventing bone loss. Several small studies have reported a higher risk of fracture among women who undergo menopause before age fifty than in those who do after age fifty.

In one study conducted by the National Institute of Child Health and

Human Development (NICHD), researchers concluded that women with primary ovarian insufficiency have a high risk of bone loss. Their findings:

- Two-thirds of the women they studied had enough bone loss that they might be at risk of a hip fracture.
- Out of the eighty-nine women they studied, seventy-seven had osteopenia (below-normal bone density and a precursor of osteoporosis). Two of the women had full-fledged osteoporosis.
- Only ten of the women in the study had normal bone density for their age.

What's worse is that about half of the women in the study had had a bone density test done within eighteen months of their POI diagnosis—and nearly half of this group already had osteopenia. Though this study focused solely on women with POI, the outlook is similar for women who are in premature menopause due to surgery or cancer treatment. Many studies indicate that if your ovaries are removed, you will experience significant bone loss in the first two years after surgery. In general, the time not on hormone replacement is significantly related to lower bone density in young women with estrogen insufficiency.

BONE TESTING

My mom has osteoporosis, and so I went and had a DEXA scan done out of pocket. I didn't have the energy at that point to argue with my GP over this issue, and I think it only cost me $250. The results I am still not that sure about. All I know is that different machines produce different readings and that there are certain brackets which indicate osteopenia and above that osteoporosis. Nobody really ever sat down with me and explained much. So I paid for this test, and I don't even know what it means.

—Erica

Diagnosing low bone density as early as possible is important because osteoporosis is a condition that can progress silently over a long period of time. Various X-rays and other tests are used to detect skeletal problems.

For some people, their health care provider might order a bone scan. Sometimes this term is incorrectly used to describe a bone density test. A bone scan involves injecting the patient with dye that allows the doctor to detect cancer, bone lesions, inflammation, or new fractures.

Some doctors might recommend a regular X-ray. However, because an X-ray can detect bone loss only after about 30 percent of the skeleton has been depleted, it is not a useful tool for detecting osteoporosis.

FACTORS THAT INCREASE YOUR RISK FOR OSTEOPOROSIS

Factors that will increase the risk of developing osteoporosis are:

- Caucasian or Asian race
- Thin, small body frames
- A family history of osteoporosis (for example, having a mother with an osteoporotic hip fracture doubles your risk of hip fracture)
- Personal history of fracture as an adult
- Cigarette smoking
- Excessive alcohol consumption
- Lack of exercise
- A diet low in calcium
- Poor nutrition and poor general health
- Malabsorption (nutrients are not properly absorbed from the gastrointestinal system) from conditions such as celiac sprue
- Low estrogen levels (such as occur in menopause or with early surgical removal of both ovaries)
- Chronic inflammation due to diseases such as rheumatoid arthritis and chronic liver diseases
- Immobility, such as after a stroke or due to any condition that interferes with walking
- Hyperthyroidism, a condition in which too much thyroid hormone is produced by the thyroid gland (as in Graves' disease) or that is caused by taking too much thyroid hormone medication
- The long-term use of certain medications, including heparin (a blood thinner), the antiseizure medications phenytoin (Dilantin) and phenobarbital, and oral corticosteroids (such as prednisone).

A bone mineral density (BMD) test is the best way to evaluate your bone health. A BMD test can accurately identify osteoporosis, your risk for fractures, and your response to your osteoporosis treatment. The most widely used BMD test is called dual-energy X-ray absorptiometry, or the DEXA test.

It measures the bone density at your hip and spine and is one of the most accurate ways to diagnose bone loss. This test is so accurate that your follow-up DEXA scan can be used to monitor your treatment to learn if it is working. The good news is that it's painless and feels a lot like having an X-ray.

DEXA scans

- Are more accurate than regular X-rays. A person would need to lose 20 to 30 percent of her bone density before it would show up on an X-ray.
- Require less radiation exposure than a CAT scan or radiographic absorptiometry. In fact, you are exposed to more radiation on a cross-country flight than you are during a DEXA scan.
- Should be performed on the same machine every time to allow for accurate comparison of results.
- Cost about $250.

This is a noninvasive test and requires very little preparation. If you are taking calcium supplements, stop taking them for forty-eight hours before your test. If you are taking any medications for osteopenia or osteoporosis, do not take them the day of your test. You can eat and drink normally on the day of the test. Some insurance companies will pay for the test, especially if you have any of the risk factors.

OSTEOPENIA OR OSTEOPOROSIS?

Osteoporosis, according to the National Osteoporosis Foundation (www .nof.com), is a disease in which bones become fragile and more likely to break. If not prevented or if left untreated, osteoporosis can progress painlessly until a bone breaks. These breaks, or fractures, typically occur in the hip, spine, and wrist.

Osteopenia is the term for low bone density that is not yet low enough to be called osteoporosis.

As with all X-rays, you should wear loose, comfortable clothing, avoiding garments that have zippers, belts, or buttons made of metal. Objects such as keys or a wallet that would be in the area being scanned should be removed. You may be asked to remove some or all of your clothes and to wear a gown during the exam. You may also be asked to remove jewelry, eyeglasses, and any metal objects or clothing that might interfere with the X-ray images. If you are pregnant, it is important to discuss the risks to the fetus with your physician and the radiologist performing the test.

The Radiological Society of North America describes the procedure in this way: In the central DEXA examination, which measures bone density in the hip and spine, the patient lies on a padded table. An X-ray generator is located below the patient, and an imaging device, or detector, is positioned above. To assess the spine, the patient's legs are supported on a padded box to flatten the pelvis and lower (lumbar) spine. To assess the hip, the patient's foot is placed in a brace that rotates the hip inward. In both cases, the detector is slowly passed over the area, generating images on a computer monitor.

You must hold very still and may be asked to stop breathing for a few seconds while the X-ray picture is taken, to reduce the possibility of a blurred image. The technologist will walk behind a wall or into the next room to activate the X-ray machine.

The DEXA machine sends a thin, invisible beam of low-dose X-rays with two distinct energy peaks through the bones being examined. One peak is absorbed mainly by soft tissue and the other by bone. The soft-tissue amount is subtracted from the total, and what remains is the patient's bone mineral density. DEXA machines feature special software that compute and display the bone density measurements on a computer monitor. The results are given to your physician, who can discuss them with you within a few days.

TEST RESULTS

Whether it's blood work, X-rays, or other lab work, always ask for a copy of the results for your own files. Doctors often tell you that test results are "normal," without giving you other information. It can be helpful to see the results, especially if your DEXA scan shows the image with the light spots that show a lack of bone density. Besides, it allows you to compare results from year to year and might be a good motivator for you. The test results are given as follows.

BONE MINERAL DENSITY First, the column marked **BMD** gives your bone mineral density, or the number of grams per centimeter of bone. A number of +1.0 or above is good.

T SCORE The T score compares the patient's bone mineral density with the mean peak bone density of a thirty-year-old person of the same sex and is expressed as a number of standard deviations above or below the young person's density. The results can be normal or defined as osteopenia or osteoporosis. The World Health Organization created the following categories based on bone density in white women:

- **Normal:** Normal bone density is when the T score is greater than −1.0.
- **At risk:** If the bone mineral density is between −1.0 and −2.5, it indicates the presence of osteopenia.
- **Serious:** If the bone mineral density is −2.5 or less, it indicates the presence of osteoporosis at the site of measurement.

Z SCORE Your Z score is the number of standard deviations above or below what's normally expected for someone of your age, sex, weight, and racial or ethnic origin.

POSSIBLE INTERFERENCE
Be sure to tell your doctor beforehand if you've recently had an oral contrast or nuclear medicine test. These tests require an injection of radioactive tracers that might interfere with your bone density test.

QUANTITATIVE COMPUTERIZED TOMOGRAPHY (QCT) SCAN

This test uses a computerized tomography (CT) scanner combined with computer software to determine your bone density, usually at your spine. Quantitative CT (QCT) scans provide detailed 3-D images and can take into account the effects of aging and diseases other than osteoporosis on your bones. QCT scans emit more radiation than DEXA scans do. For a QCT test, you lie on a movable table that's guided into a large tubelike area where images are taken. It typically takes less than ten minutes.

BONE HEALTH SUPPORT GROUPS

To join a support group for people with osteoporosis, contact the National Osteoporosis Foundation for information on the support group nearest to you. Call NOF's Education Department at 202-223-2226 or toll free at 800-231-4222.

PERIPHERAL TESTING

An ultrasound test done on a peripheral location, such as your heel, may predict the risk of fracture in your spine and hip as well. But because bone density tends to vary from one location to the other, a measurement taken at the heel usually isn't as accurate as a measurement taken at the spine or hip.

PROTECTION AGAINST OSTEOPOROSIS

The strategies listed here may slow bone loss, but none of them will prevent bone loss entirely. To protect against bone loss, the National Osteoporosis Foundation recommends that women who are at risk for osteoporosis:

- Get at least 1,200 mg of calcium in their diets every day. If it is not possible to get this amount through diet, take a calcium supplement. To maximize absorption, take calcium supplements with meals and in divided doses (typically 500 mg or less at one time).
- Get between 400 IU and 800 IU of vitamin D, which helps the body absorb calcium, every day.

- Participate in regular weight-bearing and muscle-building physical activity. Weight-bearing physical activity, such as walking, helps build bone strength. Activities such as yoga and tai chi help build muscle strength and improve flexibility.

WHAT PRODUCTS CONTAIN CAFFEINE, AND HOW MUCH?

Item	Milligrams of Caffeine	
	Typical	Range*
Coffee (8 fluid ounces)		
Brewed, drip method	85	65–120
Brewed, percolator	75	60–85
Decaffeinated, brewed	3	2–4
Espresso (1 fluid ounce)	40	30–50
Teas (8 fluid ounces)		
Brewed	40	20–90
Instant	28	24–31
Iced (8 fluid ounces)	25	9–50
Others		
Some soft drinks (8 fluid ounces)	24	20–40
"Energy" drinks	80	0–80
Cocoa beverage (8 fluid ounces)	6	3–32
Chocolate milk beverage (8 fluid ounces)	5	2–7
Milk chocolate (1 ounce)	6	1–15
Dark chocolate, semisweet (1 ounce)	20	5–35
Baker's chocolate (1 ounce)	26	26
Chocolate-flavored syrup (1 fluid ounce)	4	4

* For the coffee and tea products, the range varies due to brewing method, plant variety, brand of product, and other factors.
Source: U.S. Food and Drug Administration and National Soft Drink Association.

CAFFEINE AND BONE HEALTH

There have been many studies of caffeine and bone health, some showing that caffeine increases the risk of hip fracture and some that it has no effect. Many factors affect bone health, but it is known that caffeine increases the amount of calcium lost in urine. It also appears that a high caffeine intake (more than 300 mg per day) is a problem mainly for women who have a low calcium intake. So, to be safe, keep your caffeine intake down and your calcium intake adequate.

Dairy products are among the best sources of calcium based on their:

- Calcium content
- Absorption
- Content of other essential nutrients
- Low cost relative to total nutritional value

Approximately three cups per day of dairy products provide the 1,200-mg target.

Source: North American Menopause Society.

PRESCRIPTIONS FOR GOOD BONE HEALTH

There are a number of prescription medications on the market for the management of osteoporosis. Estrogen therapy can prevent the largest loss of bone mass that women experience. Medications containing estrogen can increase bone density by as much as 5 percent. For women who can't take estrogen or for whom estrogen is not enough, other medications such as Evista, Fosamax, and Miacalcin are available. These medications have also been shown to slow bone loss and reduce the risk of fractures. A few newer studies have suggested that there may be a connection between taking statins (typically used for lowering cholesterol) and increasing bone density. However, more research is still needed to determine the role and benefits of taking statins to reduce the risk of fractures. Overall, it is important for women with ovarian insufficiency and low estrogen levels to focus on bone health and talk to a health care provider regularly about continuous management.

Oral Health and Periodontal Disease

Changes in hormone levels can make women more susceptible to the progression of periodontitis during certain times in their lives. Ovarian insufficiency is one of those times. To prevent periodontal disease, brush your teeth at least twice daily and floss at least once daily. Have your teeth cleaned professionally twice a year if you do not have gum disease, three or four times a year if you have been diagnosed with periodontal disease. This will reduce the incidence of periodontal problems and the severity of some non-plaque-associated diseases of the mouth (i.e., lichen planus).

More frequent professional cleanings are the first line of defense to prevent such problems both because the teeth are cleaned more often and also because your periodontal status can be monitored more closely, thus reducing the likelihood that dramatic changes in your periodontal status will go unnoticed.

"My best advice is to institute a preventive dental care plan that involves a thorough understanding of [a patient's] own personal periodontal status. I encourage patients to ask questions, take ownership of what their level of health is, and try to understand what is going on in their mouth," says Eduardo R. Lorenzana, D.D.S., M.S.

DENTAL HEALTH ASSESSMENT TIP
An easy bit of information to become familiar with is when the dentist or hygienist uses the periodontal probe to measure your pockets at their cleaning visit (it should be done at least once per year). You should be aware that low numbers (less than 4 mm) are best and that the presence of high numbers (more than 4 mm) should elicit a discussion about what should be done or changed to address the problem.

"Watch and wait" is not a dental intervention strategy. Research shows that the earlier treatment is instituted, the easier it is to arrest problems and prevent their recurrence. Oral hygiene instruction and follow-through at home are critical, as are regular cleanings two to four times a year, depending on the level of severity of the periodontal condition. If treatment at your family dentist's office does not control the problem, your dentist should refer you to a periodontist. Periodontists are specialists in the treatment of advanced diseases of the gums, bone, and supporting structures of the teeth. Having excellent oral health as a foundation can minimize and potentially eliminate the development of some other, more serious, health conditions. There is no better treatment than prevention.

Oral changes in women with ovarian insufficiency may include dry mouth; pain and burning sensations in the gums, cheeks, or tongue; or altered sense of taste. In addition, a condition called desquamative gingivitis, in which the gums turn bright red, become fragile, then peel off and leave a raw, bleeding surface, is more prevalent. Such changes are brought about by the decrease in the production of sex hormones, primarily progesterone and estrogen. New research is finding that bone loss due to osteoporosis is associated with increased severity of periodontal disease. Women considering hormone therapy to prevent osteoporosis should note that similar beneficial effects have been found when studying its relationship to periodontal health. HT has been found to be protective in terms of tooth loss and decreased incidence of gingival bleeding, according to Eduardo R. Lorenzana.

Find Support

I've not been dealing with my diagnosis that well and did not have the guts to contact anyone. I was feeling very alone and didn't want to expose myself. It is not very nice having to take an HT tablet on the morning of your wedding, with your pregnant bridesmaid helping you get ready. I finally feel as though getting involved in a patient group is the only way I can start to move on and come to terms with this.

—Tina

A number of nonprofit groups offer additional resources, online chats, forums, and support groups. Online support groups and information can be found at:

- Rachel's Well, www.rachelswell.org
- The International Premature Ovarian Failure Association (IPOFA), www.pofsupport.org

- The Daisy Network, www.daisynetwork.org.uk, in the United Kingdom
- Hyster Sisters, www.hystersisters.com, for those undergoing a hysterectomy

Besides connecting with people going through similar experiences, these patient groups are also excellent resources for conferences, clinical studies, and new research results.

LOOK IT UP

The National Library of Medicine (NLM) is the world's largest medical library. Its services include PubMed, which contains publication information and (in most cases) brief summaries of articles from scientific and medical journals. NLM also maintains DIRLINE, a database that contains locations and descriptive information about a variety of health organizations.

Web site: www.nlm.nih.gov
PubMed: www.ncbi.nlm.nih.gov/entrez/
DIRLINE: http://dirline.nlm.nih.gov

Clinical Studies and New Treatments

Although there are many definitions of clinical trials, they are generally considered to be biomedical or health-related research studies in human beings that follow a predefined protocol. There are two major types of clinical trials that help researchers better understand diseases. Interventional studies are those in which the research subjects are assigned by the investigator to a treatment or other intervention and their outcomes are measured. Observational studies are those in which individuals are observed and their outcomes are measured by the investigators.

Choosing to participate in a clinical trial that focuses on ovarian insufficiency is an important personal decision. The following frequently asked questions provide detailed information about clinical trials. In addition, it is often helpful to talk to a physician, family members, or friends about deciding to join a trial. After identifying some options, the next step is to contact the study research staff and ask questions about specific trials.

WHY PARTICIPATE IN
A CLINICAL TRIAL?

Participants in clinical trials can play a more active role in their own health care, gain access to new research treatments before they are widely available, and help others by contributing to medical research.

WHO CAN PARTICIPATE IN
A CLINICAL TRIAL?

Before joining a clinical trial, a participant must qualify for the study. All clinical trials have guidelines about who can participate. The factors that allow someone to participate in a clinical trial are called "inclusion criteria," and those that disallow someone from participating are called "exclusion criteria." These criteria are based on such factors as age, gender, the type and stage of a disease, previous treatment history, and other medical conditions. Some research studies seek participants with illnesses or conditions to be studied in the clinical trial, while others need healthy participants. It is important to note that inclusion and exclusion criteria are not used to reject people personally. Instead, they are used to identify appropriate participants and keep them safe. The criteria help ensure that researchers will be able to answer the questions they plan to study.

WHAT ARE THE BENEFITS AND RISKS OF
PARTICIPATING IN A CLINICAL TRIAL?

Clinical trials that are well designed and well executed are the best way for an eligible participant to:

- Play an active role in her own health care
- Gain access to new research treatments before they are widely available
- Obtain expert medical care at leading health care facilities during the trial
- Help others by contributing to medical research
- Save money by accessing potentially free medical treatment, medicines, and so on.

There are, however, risks associated with clinical trials:

- Experimental treatments may have unpleasant, serious, or even life-threatening side effects.
- The experimental treatment may not be effective for an individual participant.
- The protocol may require more of a patient's time and attention than would a nonprotocol treatment, including trips to the study site, more treatments, hospital stays, or complex dosage requirements.

LOCATE CLINICAL TRIALS
Center Watch www.centerwatch.com
Clinical Trials www.clinicaltrials.gov
Women's Health Initiative www.whi.org

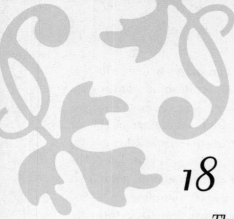

18

The Future of Care

My diagnosis was unexpected and unwelcomed. Nevertheless, my POF has had a strange, uplifting effect on my life. I now recognize the importance of life and what a gift it truly is. Every day that goes by, I am thankful for being alive. Every day that goes by, I am thankful for my son. Don't get me wrong, like probably all women with this, every day that goes by, I continue to wish that my diagnosis could be reversed. Yes, I still long and wish for the ability to have another biological child. Yes, I worry constantly about my hormone levels, my bone loss, my early aging, and all the other things that come with POI. But I now see every day as a learning day. I continually search for new ways to deal with my illness, and I will continually work on my HT regimen (which needs to be routinely updated and refined). POI is not something that I can change or cure, so I am learning to live with it in the best possible way.

—Kaye

The Future of Research

Currently, many researchers, including those at the National Institutes of Health (NIH), are conducting and sponsoring a number of studies on POI, such as:

- Exploring whether a low dose of a certain steroid, prednisone, can treat POI in cases caused by an autoimmune disorder. The steroid decreases the function of the body's immune system, which is thought to be attacking the ovary follicles in some women with POI.

- Trying to determine the best combination and dosage of HT for treating POI. Some researchers are trying to learn whether adding testosterone to a woman's HT can help to prevent bone loss. Others are trying to find the amount of estrogen and progestin that will best treat POI without causing too many side effects.
- Focusing on what happens in an ovary that is working normally. This information may help scientists develop a test for early detection of POI.

Clinical trials to explore these topics are already under way. To find out more about current studies, contact the NIH Patient Recruitment and Public Liaison Office at 1-800-411-1222. You can also learn more about all studies on POI by going to http://clinicaltrials.gov, and doing a search for "premature ovarian failure."

The Future of Fertility Preservation

Because fertility is an important concern for women with diminished ovarian function, many wonder if there are opportunities to restore their fertility or prevent their reproductive capacity from decreasing any more. Unfortunately, these types of options are not available yet. With more attention paid to ovarian insufficiency as well as to the millions of women affected, it is hopeful that researchers will begin to better understand how to preserve women's fertility. Researchers are looking at ways to reverse high levels of FSH, combat low levels of estrogen, and maximize ovarian reserve.

One new method for fertility preservation that has gained a lot of notoriety lately is the possibility of transplanting ovaries. It makes sense—if you can successfully transplant other organs, why not the ovary?

The first live birth resulting from an ovary transplant occurred in London in 2008. The woman's ovaries stopped working when she was fifteen, and she became pregnant a year after receiving a donor ovary from her identical twin sister. Obviously, having a twin sister to donate an ovary means the eggs are the same genetically. For most patients, it is simpler and significantly less expensive to have IVF with donor eggs. However, the surgery would allow for the possibility of removing and freezing an ovary prior to cancer treatment such as radiotherapy and chemotherapy.

Advocacy Opportunities

The diagnosis of any type of ovarian disfunction can bring many changes and challenges. We each deal with challenges in our own way, and ovarian insufficiency is no exception. If in the course of reading this book you have seen things that you may be able to focus on or change, it might be a good time to have a go at it. If you need help for depression, anxiety, or low self-esteem, it can be very valuable to talk to someone, such as a friend or health professional, even if only once. Sharing your thoughts with people who understand, such as a support group, can be helpful also. Most important, it is helpful to take action to deal with the emotional changes, so try talking, writing in a journal, art therapy such as painting or drawing, or some form of physical activity. Taking action and seeking help can enable you to feel more informed and more in control and find strategies for coping with the changes of an ovarian insufficiency.

Menstrual Cycle Symptom Tracker

Rank symptoms on scale:

0—Not present; **1**—Symptom is present, but not that bad; **2**—Fair; **3**—Bad; **4**—Unbearable

MENSTRUAL CYCLE DIARY

Cycle Day	1	2	3	4	5	6	7	8	9	10	11	12	13	14	15	16	17	18	19	20	21	22	23	24	25	26	27	28
Date																												

SYMPTOMS

Menstrual

| Blood flow | | | | | | | | | | | | | | | | | | | | | | | | | | | | |
| Pain/ cramps | | | | | | | | | | | | | | | | | | | | | | | | | | | | |

Emotional

| Irritability | | | | | | | | | | | | | | | | | | | | | | | | | | | | |
| Moodiness | | | | | | | | | | | | | | | | | | | | | | | | | | | | |

Angry
oubursts

Poor
impulse
control

Tension or
anxiety

Depression

Lethargy

Insomnia

Crying

Social
withdrawa

Loss of
concentration,
confusion

MENSTRUAL CYCLE SYMPTOM TRACKER (CONTINUED)

Cycle Day	1	2	3	4	5	6	7	8	9	10	11	12	13	14	15	16	17	18	19	20	21	22	23	24	25	26	27	28
Date																												
Physical																												
Bloating																												
Weight increase																												
Increased appetite																												
Breast pain or tenderness																												
Skin problems																												
Hot flashes/ night sweats																												
Headache																												

Dizziness, poor
concentration,
clumsiness

Changes in libido
or sexual desire

Changes in
urination or
bowel habits

Increased thirst

Menstrual History Questionnaire

Questions to Discuss with Your Health Care Provider

- How old were you when you had your first period (menarche)?
- What were your periods like as a teenager?
- What menstruation-related symptoms did you experience as a teenager?
- When was the first day of your last period?
- How long is your typical period?
- How regular are your periods? What are the shortest and longest times between periods?
- Have you experienced spells of no periods?
- How heavy are your periods?
- How many tampons or pads do you use in a day?
- How painful are your periods?
- Do you have any bleeding between periods?
- Do you ever have bleeding after intercourse?
- What types of symptoms do you experience with your periods?
- Are you experiencing any menopause-related symptoms?

Resources

Adoption

Creating a Family
www.creatingafamily.com

**Dave Thomas Foundation
for Adoption**
www.davethomasfoundation.org

National Adoption Center
www.adopt.org

Bladder and Urinary Conditions

American Urogynecological Society
www.augs.org

**InContiNet
(Incontinence on the Internet)**
www.incontinet.org

**National Association for
Continence**
www.nafc.org

Cancer

American Cancer Society
www.cancer.org

Fertile Hope
www.fertilehope.org

LIVESTRONG SurvivorCare
www.livestrong.org/survivorcare

**The National Alliance of Breast
Cancer Organizations**
www.nabco.org

Complementary and Alternative Medicine

Alternative Medicine Foundation
www.amfoundation.org

**NIH National Center for
Complementary and Alternative
Medicine**
www.nccam.nih.gov

Depression

**Depression and Bipolar Support
Alliance (DBSA)**
www.dbsalliance.org

Mental Health America
www.nmha.org

Fertility

American Fertility Association
www.theafa.org

The American Society for Reproductive Medicine
www.asrm.org

Choice Moms
www.choicemoms.org

My Fertility Plan
www.myfertilityplan.com

Resolve: The National Infertility Association
www.resolve.org

Fragile X Research and Information

National Fragile X Foundation
www.fragilex.org

Galactosemia and Turner's Syndrome

Parents of Galactosemic Children, Inc.
www.galactosemia.org

Turner Syndrome Society of the United States
www.turner-syndrome-us.org

Genetic Information

Genetic Alliance
www.geneticalliance.org

National Society of Genetic Counselors
www.nsgc.org

Your Genes, Your Health
www.ygyh.org

Heart Disease

American Heart Association
www.americanheart.org

Hormones

The Hormone Foundation
www.hormone.org

Lesbian Health

Gay and Lesbian Medical Association
www.glma.org

The National Women's Health Information Center
www.womenshealth.gov/faq/lesbian-health.cfm

Menopause

The Alexander Foundation for Women's Health
www.afwh.org

American Menopause Foundation
www.americanmenopause.org

The European Menopause and Andropause Society
www.emas-online.org

North American Menopause Society
www.menopause.org

ProjectAWARE
www.project-aware.org

Osteoporosis

National Osteoporosis Foundation
www.nof.org

Premature Ovarian Failure/Primary Ovarian Insufficiency

Daisy Network Premature Menopause Support Group
www.daisynetwork.org.uk

International Premature Ovarian Failure Association
www.pofsupport.org

Rachel's Well
www.rachelswell.org

Sexuality

American Association of Sexuality Educators Counselors & Therapists
www.aasect.org

International Academy of Sex Research
www.iasr.org

International Society for the Study of Women's Sexual Health
www.isswsh.org

Sex Information and Education Council of Canada
www.sieccan.org

The Society for the Scientific Study of Sexuality
www.sexscience.org

The Women's Sexual Health Foundation
www.twshf.org

Sleep

National Sleep Foundation
www.sleepfoundation.org

Weight Control

NIH Weight-Control Information Network
http://win.niddk.nih.gov

Shape Up America
http://shapeup.org

Women's Health (General)

Jean Hailes Foundation
www.jeanhailes.org.au

National Research Center for Women & Families
www.center4research.org/womenhlth1.html

National Women's Health Information Center
www.womenshealth.gov

National Women's Health Network
www.nwhn.org

National Women's Health Research Center
www.healthywoman.org

Our Bodies Ourselves
www.ourbodiesourselves.org

Books

ADOPTION

Davenport, Dawn. *The Complete Book of International Adoption: A Step by Step Guide to Finding Your Child.* New York: Broadway, 2006.

Falker, Elizabeth Swire. *The Ultimate Insider's Guide to Adoption.* New York: Wellness Central, 2006.

BLADDER AND URINARY CONDITIONS

Hulme, Janet A. *Beyond Kegels: Fabulous Four Exercises & More to Prevent & Treat Incontinence.* Blaine, Wash.: Phoenix Publishing, 2006.

Parker, William. *The Incontinence Solution: Answers for Women of All Ages.* New York: Fireside, 2002.

CANCER

Del Priore, Giuseppe, and J. Richard Smith. *Women's Cancers: Pathways to Healing: A Patients Guide to Dealing with Ovarian and Breast Cancer.* New York: Springer, 2009.

Hartmann, Lynn C., and Charles L. Loprinzi. *Mayo Clinic Guide to Women's Cancers.* Rochester, Minn.: Mayo Clinic, 2005.

CARDIAC HEALTH

Goldberg, Nieca. *The Women's Healthy Heart Program: Lifesaving Strategies for Preventing and Healing Heart Disease.* New York: Ballantine, 2006.

Samaan, Sarah. *The Smart Woman's Guide to Heart Health: Dr. Sarah's Seven Steps to a Heart-Loving Lifestyle.* Dallas, Tex.: Brown Books, 2009.

von der Lohe, Elizabeth. *Coronary Heart Disease in Women: Prevention, Diagnosis, Therapy.* New York: Springer, 2003.

DEPRESSION

Hart, Archibald, and Catherine Hart Weber. *Unveiling Depression in Women: A Practical Guide to Understanding and Overcoming Depression.* Grand Rapids, Mich.: Revell, 2001.

———. *Woman's Guide to Overcoming Depression.* Grand Rapids, Mich.: Revell, 2007.

FERTILITY

Glazer, Elen Sarasohn, and Evelina Weidman Sterling. *Having Your Baby Through Egg Donation.* Indianapolis, Ind.: Perspectives Press, 2000.

Sterling, Evelina, and Angie Best-Boss. *Budgeting for Infertility: Bringing Home Baby Without Breaking the Bank.* New York: Fireside, 2009.

HORMONES

Rako, Susan. *The Hormone of Desire: The Truth About Testosterone, Sexuality & Menopause.* New York: Three Rivers Press, 1999.

COMPLEMENTARY AND ALTERNATIVE MEDICINE

Hudson, Tori. *Women's Encyclopedia of Natural Medicine: Alternative Therapies and Integrative Medicine for Total Health and Wellness.* Columbus, Ohio: McGraw-Hill, 2007.

Ojeda, Linda, and Jeffrey S. Bland. *Menopause Without Medicine: The Trusted Women's Resource with the Latest Information on HRT, Breast Cancer, Heart Disease, and Natural Estrogens.* Alameda, Calif.: Hunter House, 2003.

LESBIAN HEALTH

Kerr, Shelly, and Robin M. Mathy. *Preventive Health Measures for Lesbian and Bisexual Women.* London: Informa Health Care, 2007.

White, Jocelyn. *The Lesbian Health Book.* Berkeley, Calif.: Seal Press, 1997.

MENOPAUSE

Boston Women's Health Book Collective, Judy Norsigian, and Vivian Pinn. *Our Bodies, Ourselves: Menopause.* New York: Touchstone, 2006.

Keegan, Leslie. *Mind Over Menopause: The Complete Mind/Body Approach to Coping with Menopause.* New York: Free Press, 2004.

Landau, Carol, and Michele G. Cyr. *The New Truth About Menopause: Straight Talk About Treatments and Choices from Two Leading Women Doctors.* New York: St. Martin's Press, 2003.

Watson, Cynthia M. *User's Guide to Easing Menopause Symptoms Naturally: Learn How to Prevent Hot Flashes and Other Symptoms Safely and Naturally.* Laguna Beach, Calif.: Basic Health Publications, 2003.

NUTRITION

Pensiero, Laura J., Michael P. Osborne, and Susan Oliveria. *The Strang Cancer Prevention Center Cookbook.* Columbus, Ohio: McGraw-Hill, 2008.

OSTEOPOROSIS

Cosman, Felicia. *What Your Doctor May Not Tell You About Osteoporosis: Help Prevent—and Even Reverse—the Disease That Burdens Millions of Women.* New York: Warner Books, 2003.

Gates, Ronda, Beverly Whipple, and Florence Henderson. *Smart Women, Strong Bones.* Winchester, Wash.: Lifestyles Press, 2000.

Miriam, Nelson, and Sarah Wernick. *Strong Women, Strong Bones.* New York: Perigee, 2006.

PREMATURE OVARIAN FAILURE

POF Support Group. *Faces of POF: Learning and Living with Premature Ovarian Failure.* Alexandria, Va.: International Premature Ovarian Failure Support Group, Inc., 2004.

SEXUALITY

Hall, Kathryn. *Reclaiming Your Sexual Self: How You Can Bring Desire Back into Your Life.* Hoboken, N.J.: Wiley, 2004.

Love, Patricia. *Hot Monogamy: Essential Steps to More Passionate, Intimate Lovemaking.* New York: Plume Books, 1995.

SLEEP

Epstein, Lawrence, and Steven Mardon. *The Harvard Medical School Guide to a Good Night's Sleep.* Columbus, Ohio: McGraw-Hill, 2006.

Kinosian, Janet. *The Well-rested Woman: 60 Soothing Suggestions for Getting a Good Night's Sleep.* Newburyport, Mass.: Conari Press, 2000.

Weil, Andrew. *Healthy Sleep: Fall Asleep Easily, Sleep More Deeply, Sleep Through the Night, Wake Up Refreshed* (audiobook). Louisville, Colo.: Sounds True, 2007.

WOMEN'S HEALTH

Boston Women's Health Book Collective. *Our Bodies, Ourselves.* New York: Touchstone, 2005.

Sparrowe, Linda. *The Woman's Book of Yoga and Health: A Lifelong Guide to Wellness.* Boston, Mass.: Shambhala, 2002.

Acknowledgments

Every book is the creation of more than its authors. We have been fortunate to work with many gifted and collaborative colleagues, including Marcie Richardson, M.D.; Valerie Baker, M.D.; Lawrence Nelson, M.D.; Karin A. Clark, M.A.; The North American Menopause Society; Eduardo R. Lorenzana, D.D.S.; Robert Rebar, M.D.; Paula Hillard, M.D.; Benjamin Leader; M.D., Ph.D.; and Sharon Covington, M.S.W.

We thank Rebekah Worthman for her editing, as well as Emily Klinedinst, Kaylyn Boss, and our families, for whom we are grateful.

The book would not be in existence without the help and encouragement of our agent, Susanna Einstein. Michelle Howry, our editor at Touchstone, and her team once again made this book better with their careful guidance and rigorous scrutiny.

Index

About the Authors

Evelina Weidman Sterling

Evelina is an accomplished and well-known infertility expert, public health educator, and researcher. She is the CEO of My Fertility Plan (www.myfertilityplan.com), a leading infertility consulting firm aimed at providing health care consumers and infertility patients with a wide range of unbiased and evidence-based educational resources and referrals. My Fertility Plan helps patients better navigate through their fertility care and encourages informed decision making.

Evelina has cowritten several other best-selling and award-winning books focusing on reproductive health, including *Living with Polycystic Ovary Syndrome* (Addicus Books, 2000) and *Having Your Baby through Egg Donation* (Perspectives Press, 2005). She has also published several articles and has given numerous interviews and presentations about various aspects of fertility, including the many complex issues associated with overcoming infertility.

She holds a Ph.D. in medical sociology from Georgia State University as well as a master's degree in public health from the Johns Hopkins University. She also attended the University of Mary Washington, where she earned a bachelor of science degree in biology. Evelina has over fifteen years' experience working in public health education and research, primarily in the areas of reproductive and women's health. Previous experience includes positions at Healthy Mothers, Healthy Babies National Coalition; American Association for Health Education; Health Resources and Services Administration, Gallaudet University; and the American Heart Association. She also regularly serves as an independent consultant helping nonprofit organizations and government agencies effectively develop, implement, and evaluate public health and health education programs. Currently, she is serving as president of Rachel's Well, an innovative nonprofit organization that promotes more research and education in women's health, particularly focusing on primary ovarian insufficiency and menstrual health.

Evelina is passionate and committed to providing all families with the tools they need to grow their families. She lives in Atlanta with her husband and two children.

Angie Best-Boss

Angie is an award-winning women's health writer and a passionate infertility consumer advocate. She is currently the president of My Fertility Plan (www.my fertilityplan.com). In addition to coauthoring *Living with PCOS* (Addicus Books, 2000), Angie has written three other nonfiction books, including *The Everything Guide to Digestive Health.* She has a bachelor of arts degree in sociology and journalism from Virginia Wesleyan College and a master of divinity degree with an emphasis in counseling from Union Theological Seminary.

Her articles on women's health and infertility have appeared in dozens of both online and print resources, including *MD News, Massage Therapy Today, Family Building Magazine,* www.conceivingconcepts.com, www.obgyn.net, www.iparent ing.com, and www.pcosupport.org. She is the lead medical writer for www.con ceivingconcepts.com and is a member of the American Medical Writers Association and the American Reproductive Health Professionals Association. She is a featured blogger at How to Make a Family: Baby-Making from Every Conceivable Angle (http://howtomakeafamily.typepad.com.)

Angie lives in New Palestine, Indiana, with her husband and three daughters.